Your Powerful Choice: Fighting Obesity and the Obesity Gene

Your Powerful Choice: Fighting Obesity and the Obesity Gene

Timothy Falcon Crack

*PhD (MIT), MCom, PGDipCom,
BSc (HONS 1st Class)*

Published by: Timothy Falcon Crack, P.O. Box 6385, Dunedin North, Dunedin 9059, New Zealand, Revised and Corrected Second Edition, January 2016.

ISBN: 978-0-9941182-7-1

Typeset by the author.
Printed in the U.S.A., U.K., and Australia
www.YourPowerfulChoice.com
timcrack@alum.mit.edu

Contents

CONTENTS

Introduction

This is not a complicated book. This is not a long book. There are no recipes, no menu plans, and no exercise plans. Rather, this is a book about informed decision making. It contains information, observations, and advice designed to help you make a powerful choice: the choice to attain and maintain good health and a healthy weight.

I have three goals in writing this book. First, I firmly believe that many people do not realize that they possess the power and the right to change their future outcomes for the better. So, my first goal is to give some examples from my life, to demonstrate that empowerment is an option that you can choose. In fact, once I realized how powerful my choices were, many things changed for the better in my life. I am hopeful that my experiences will help you to be able to recognize opportunities where you can choose better outcomes for yourself.

Second, I firmly believe that most doctors have zero faith in the ability of the average patient to turn their life around and make healthy choices. Maybe that's because doctors are always reading medical literature that describes the terribly unhealthy outcomes patients have inflicted upon themselves by overeating or smoking or drinking to excess, etc. So, they look down upon most people as being beyond redemption. It could also be that doctors face a steady stream of unhealthy people every day, and they have simply become jaded by overexposure to people who have failed to turn their lives around.

Whatever the reason, doctors often choose not to pass on unpopular facts and figures that could help you choose to change your lifestyle. So, I want to do exactly that: To pass on facts and figures so that you can make educated decisions. If you educate yourself and then you still choose to be unhealthy, at least it will be an informed decision, not an uninformed one.

Note that I often cite recent research articles to back up my facts and figures. Full details for these citations appear in the references section.

Third, empowerment and education are fine, but they are not enough. You also need techniques to bring about change in your life. So, I want to share with you the mental and physical techniques that proved successful for me. I was able to use these techniques to fight a very strong genetic predisposition towards obesity, to get to a healthy weight, and to maintain that healthy weight for over 30 years. I am hopeful that sharing these techniques will help you to achieve similar outcomes. Note that you will have to be honest with yourself and with your friends and family if you are to succeed.

If you benefit from the contents of this book, as I have benefited from them, then I am interested in hearing from you and potentially including a summary of your success story in a revised edition of this book, and/or on my Web site, with your permission. Please put "Your Powerful Choice" in the subject line of your email, be brief, and allow several weeks for a response.

Finally, if after reading this book and making the sorts of personal choices I describe, you find that your health and quality of life improves, then I invite you to go to Amazon.com and leave a positive review for this book so that other people may similarly benefit from it. Just type the ISBN number from the back cover into Amazon's Web site and then click on the box labeled "Write a customer review." Thank you.

TFC/2016

www.YourPowerfulChoice.com
timcrack@alum.mit.edu

Chapter 1

You Get to Choose

This book is called "Your Powerful Choice" because it is about *empowering choices*. It is about recognizing, accepting, and embracing the fact that you have the right and the ability to choose healthy outcomes. Your choices are powerful, and you can be empowered by your choices.

I want to make three points in this chapter: first, in many situations during your life, you get to choose outcomes for yourself; second, I believe many people fail to recognize these opportunities to choose outcomes, and unfortunately these opportunities then pass them by; and third, once you can recognize opportunities to choose outcomes, you are empowered to change your life. Let me explain.

One of the most important things I have learned in my life is that in many cases I got to choose outcomes for myself. My repeated experience has been, however, that nobody ever told me what my choices were, or that the choices were mine to make. I had to figure it out for myself by trial and error.

I want to share with you my personal approach to fighting weight gain. It made such a dramatic/profound difference to my life that I am hopeful that it can help you too. In fact, I am angry that nobody told me sooner that these choices existed and that it was my right to make them. You should be angry too.

I do not claim to have a solution that will work for everyone. I chose a path and followed it; your path will be different, suited to your strengths and weaknesses. I consider myself lucky to be at an extremely disciplined person because my discipline allowed me to conquer multiple very difficult challenges. I admit that on occasion maybe I went too far in challenging myself, but along the way I learned some useful techniques for meeting difficult goals.

You may have more modest goals than I had. Maybe you are 300 pounds and you just want to get down to 225 and be able to walk around the block with your spouse (never mind getting down to 175 and being able to go jogging).

You may have no real confidence in your ability to fight your weight gain. Your doctor, your friends, and even your family may have given up on your ability to change your life. I have confidence, however, that you can succeed in getting healthy, or at least that you can become much healthier than you are now. I believe that once you are empowered, you can achieve great outcomes for yourself. So, this chapter is all about empowerment.

I was the largest of five babies in my family. I was a plump toddler, a chubby child/teenager, and a fat young man. Yes, *fat*. Don't call it anything else. Don't say "heavy," or "overweight," or "big," or anything else. I was *fat*. You are *fat*.

Let me explain something really important here. I can make no apologies for using the word "fat" repeatedly in this book. It is a simple statement of scientific truth. It was not until I openly and honestly labeled myself as "fat" that I reached a turning point in my life. I found it *liberating* to admit that I was fat, that I had a problem, and that I had to do something about it. It was like a breath of fresh air to be so honest and open about something previously not even spoken about.

If you find the "fat" label offensive, then I urge you to reconsider your views because I don't think you are being honest about your issues. I was in your shoes and in your head and I know how important honesty is. Calling a spade a spade is part of that. **So, you have to be honest with yourself, your friends, and your family.**

Let me continue. I was the fat kid in school back in the 1970s when there was only one fat kid per class. I had two sisters who were, variously, overweight, obese, or morbidly obese. My mother was overweight or obese. My mother's mother and my mother's aunts were all overweight or obese. My brother and my father were, however, quite slender. So, my body fatness was inherited from my mother's side, rather than being environmental. I have to say that if there is such a thing as the obesity gene (and I don't claim that there is), then I surely have it.

Although I am now slender, I still have issues. I know my body wants to be obese. For example, I am hungry all the time, I gain weight incredibly quickly, and I lose weight only agonizingly slowly. Although anybody who looks at me would think I don't have a weight issue, they would be mistaken.

I have an issue, it is just that it is under control.

Just over 30 years ago, before I was 20 years old, I was fat and unhealthy, and on a one-way road towards what appeared to be predestined obesity. I was, however, sick and tired of being fat. I hated it and I chose to fight it. Although I was strongly genetically predisposed towards obesity, I chose not to be fat any longer. Nobody told me that I had the right or the ability to make that choice; I had to figure it out for myself.

I firmly believe that choosing not to be fat any longer is a decision that you too can make. Although the basic techniques are simple to understand, they are difficult to implement. So, you have to accept now that it is going to be hard work to get healthy and stay healthy. You must be committed to your choice. **You really have to want it or it won't happen.**

Conversely, anyone who offers you an easy solution to being fat is a charlatan. Any diet where you eat whatever you want is a scam. Any diet with healthy food groups missing is a fad and a scam; it cannot be a part of the long-term road to good health. People selling these scams will take your money, and you will soon be back where you started, only poorer, and still fat.

My experience with fad diets was that I tried several different diets and none of them worked for me. On diets where other folks lost weight, I gained weight. I tried low-carb high-protein diets, but my constant hunger just loved it, and I gained weight. Someone mentioned to me recently a diet where you can eat as much fruit as you want, but it would never have worked for me; I love bananas and I would have quickly gained weight on that diet. (See further discussion of fad diets in Chapter 6.)

So, after many failed attempts, I chose to educate myself. I decided that I was smart enough to figure it out for myself, rather than listening to diet gurus whose words certainly did not seem to work for me. I went to my local hospital and got a bunch of literature from a dietician, and I borrowed books on exercise from the library.

All the education in the world is worthless to you, however, if you do not have the honesty to admit that you are unhealthy, the winning mind (see Chapter 5) needed to make a permanent commitment to a change in lifestyle, and the intestinal fortitude to stick to that change in lifestyle over the long run.

I think many people (doctors, family, friends, and perhaps you) tip-toe around important weight loss issues. You may be afraid or embarrassed to admit "I am fat" and to say it out loud. Hey, don't you think everybody knows it already? I think, on some level, you know it already too. People are afraid, however, to call a fat person a "fat person" because they think it is callous or rude.

"Fat" should not be a dirty word. Once I admitted that I was fat and unhealthy, I viewed my body fatness simply as "excess baggage" that I wanted to rid myself of. If you had come up to me and called me fat, it would have been no more offensive to me than you telling me that I have brown/green eyes, or that I look like my grandfather. It was a simple statement of fact.

(As an aside, I think the term "overweight" has to be used carefully. Overweight relative to what, or overweight relative to whom exactly? You might be overweight relative to what is a healthy weight for you, but underweight relative to your friends and family. So, much of the time in this book I just say "fat." When I am clearly talking about your weight relative to a healthy weight, however, then I will say "overweight" instead.)

If someone had come to me sooner and said "Hey, friend, you are seriously fat. You need to take ownership of your problem and do something about it," it would have been good for me, not insulting. It would have been a wakeup call. It would have been evidence that someone cared enough to state something typically not spoken out loud.

However, I think that everyone around me when I was young just assumed that because I had always been fat, and so many other people in my family tree were fat, that I too had inherited the gene for it, and I had no choice in the matter. Either nobody knew better, or nobody cared enough, or nobody was honest with me, or nobody wanted to insult me, or some combination of those causes. Whatever the cause, nobody said anything to me about my unhealthy weight, and I had to figure out for myself both that I had a choice about my weight gain and how to fight my weight gain.

This was a very dangerous situation for me to be in because if I had not had the initiative to figure it out for myself, I believe that I would certainly be morbidly obese today. So, I want to help you go through the same process of change that I was fortunate enough to go through.

The very first step is to be honest about how unhealthy you are. It is time to be sensitive to long-term health issues and to bring them to light plainly and clearly. "Make it plain," human rights activist Malcolm X would have said.

Unfortunately, we live in some sort of new world in which people are told by the media that they must bend over backwards to be accepting of other people and their differences. We are supposed to accept people for who they are or who they have chosen to be. If we make any innocent observation about anyone who is different from us in any way, we risk being targeted in the media and fired from our jobs, labeled as racist or sexist or homophobic or xenophobic or cacomorphobic (yes, there is even a name for a fear of fat people). Maybe we are none of those things. Maybe we just want to talk honestly about differences because we can use that conversation to break down barriers and learn something powerfully healthy.

I watched a current events show on television recently where a couple brought their daughter to the doctor. The daughter was maybe 12–15 years old, and she was clearly obese. The doctor examined the girl (height, weight, skin fold test, etc.), and after the examination he declared her to be obese. The mother immediately burst into tears saying that she had not known. I was surprised that she missed something so obvious. Perhaps all her daughter's school friends were the same size. Perhaps all the mother's friends were the same size. Perhaps the mother was in denial or not educated. Whatever the cause, viewing fat people as the new normal is unhealthy.

We are too accepting. It has gone too far. Doctors are afraid to tell fat people that it takes *hard work* to get to a healthy weight (nobody ever told me!). Doctors are afraid to tell fat people that there is no quick fix for obesity, that getting to a healthy weight and retraining your brain and body can take *years*, that this cannot be delivered to you in a pill or via surgery, and that you are going to need patience (nobody ever told me that either!).

Instead, all manner of ridiculous weight loss schemes are marketed to optimistic fat people who have never been told the truth. They sign up for "systems" and "packages" that will never work because they are not designed to work. It is like the band of crooks who sells you a pet pigeon, except that it turns out to be their homing pigeon, and they get to sell it to you again and again.

You have to recognize that anything that sounds too good to be true is too good to be true. **It is time to be honest. There is no easy fix for being an unhealthy weight. There is no easy fix for the obesity epidemic.**

There are many things in your life that you have no control over, but your weight is not one of them. I was fat and headed for predestined obesity, but I made the choice to reach and maintain a healthy weight. I know other people who were similarly fat, but who made the choice to reach and maintain a healthy weight, and succeeded. If I can do it, and if they can do it, then you can do it too. It is your right to choose this outcome for yourself.

Let me now give some more background material and some examples of empowering choices.

When I was a young child, my parents separated and divorced in an unpleasant, money-sucking mess that left my family dirt poor. Even the poor people had more money than us! My parents had not been to university; they lived in England during WWII, and even by 1950, U.K. university study was still roughly only one-twentieth as common as it is now as a percentage of population (Bolton, 2012). Nevertheless, I chose to go to university for an undergraduate degree, as part of the first generation of my family to ever do so. After making that choice, I also chose to graduate with no debt. So, I worked every opportunity I had to build my savings. I lived extremely frugally, and I succeeded in graduating with no debt and with modest savings.

Sure enough, university study was cheaper 25 years ago, as a proportion of average income, than it is now, but nevertheless, this was an accomplishment and I felt empowered.

So, I then chose to study more. I started postgraduate studies. My goal was not only to graduate without any debt, but to graduate with enough money to buy a house. Nobody told me this was an option, but I figured it out for myself, and I executed my choice by working full time, studying full time, and investing carefully.

I figured out that there were 168 hours in a week, so even if you study 60 hours a week, work 40 hours a week, and sleep eight hours a night, you still have a dozen hours of free time left over. It is easy to live frugally when you work that hard because you have no time to spend any money!

In practice, sleep gave way to work, and many all-nighters were required, but when I had finished with my master's degree in New Zealand (N.Z.), I had no debt and enough money saved to buy an average-priced house in my city with no mortgage.

Sure enough, real estate, like university study, was cheaper 25 years ago, as a proportion of average income, than it is now, but this was still a considerable accomplishment at that time.

More things then started to look like doors that might be open to me. So, before completing my master's degree, I applied for entry to U.S. PhD programs. Of those that accepted me, I chose to go to MIT, and then, rather than buying that house, I ended up spending half my savings supporting myself for five years while completing my PhD at MIT (I also spent a semester at the well-manicured Harvard Business School). The other half of my savings (plus a scholarship I won) meant that I was able to graduate from my PhD with money in the bank.

Nobody I knew, except my college professors, had published books, but I decided to write my first book while I was still a student at MIT. Why not? It looked like another open door. I took my book to 10 different reputable publishers, each of whom refused to publish it, telling me that it would never sell. Ignoring the criticism of others is, however, one of my strongest personality traits. So, I self-published my first book and have subsequently sold over 50,000 copies of it.

Life can deal you lousy hands beyond your control, but what matters is whether you choose to fight, and how you choose to fight. Although I came from a dirt poor, broken home in N.Z., my parents never went to college, and I was strongly genetically predisposed towards obesity, I ended up slender, relatively fit, an MIT graduate who also got to study at Harvard, and a published author. The point I am trying to make by mentioning these outcomes is that it was empowering for me to recognize that in many cases in my life, I had the right and the ability to make choices. I had to recognize the opportunities when they presented themselves. I had to ignore naysayers and grab opportunities whenever possible.

Of course, there was a certain amount of luck involved. I am lucky that I was raised in a city with a university that had a good mathematics department. I am lucky that my brain was wired to be good at mathematics, because that gave me good grades that got me into MIT. I am lucky that my brain is wired in such a way that I can ignore criticism from others and charge ahead regardless.

I am also lucky that I am at one end of the spectrum in terms of being able to take physical pain or discomfort. On that note, let me tell you one last story about making choices. I got hurt badly in an accident when I was in my early 20s. I hurt my feet, ankles, knees, one hip, and one hand. I was in extreme pain for more than six months. About nine or 10 months after the accident, I was recovered enough to begin light exercise again. It was only then that I noticed that both my feet were now pointing to about one o'clock! Darn it, I refused to stumble around like that! So, I chose to walk normally, with my feet pointed to 12 o'clock. This required considerable effort on my part and more months of pain, but I ended up walking relatively normally. Life dealt me another lousy hand, but I chose to fight.

Whether it was graduating without debt, completing a PhD at MIT, or forcing my body to walk normally after a bad accident, arriving at that outcome was simple, but not easy. It took commitment and hard work, and, in many cases, an element of luck. I recognized, accepted, and embraced the fact that I had the power and the right to choose how I lived my life. I then figured out how to execute my wishes and followed through. It was all about empowerment regarding choices on the one hand, and educated strategies for exercising those choices on the other.

Similarly, I woke up one day and I chose not to be fat any more. I was sick of it. After making that choice, I had to educate myself in order to exercise my choice. In the next chapter I discuss five simple truths that resulted from that education.

Chapter 2

Five Simple Truths

Let me now share five simple truths that I figured out by myself that have been a key to my having obtained a healthy weight.

First and foremost, weight loss is not the goal. My guess is that you have been trying to lose weight for quite some time. I tried that too, suckered in by all the misinformation out there about weight loss. When I tried to lose weight, everything I tried failed. Some of my attempts even led to my *gaining* weight. Has that been your experience too?

That's because the correct goal is not *to lose weight* but *to get healthy*, and by getting healthy, you achieve a *healthy weight*. I will explain more in the following chapters. For now, accept that aiming at weight loss as your goal has not worked for you (or me) in the past and is unlikely to work in the future; it is the wrong goal.

Second, your body is a machine. It is a complicated biological machine, but it is a machine nevertheless. If you put 2,000 calories into your body, and you burn 2,500 calories, then this negative energy gap means that you must lose weight. If you put 2,500 calories into your body, and you burn 2,000 calories, then this positive energy gap means that you must gain weight.

Sure enough, different types of calories can alter your well-being in different ways. Some empty calories are likely to leave you hungry very soon, and junk food may be unsatisfying and give you a sugar rush, etc., but the simple fact remains that your body is a machine and you need to understand body arithmetic. That's what Chapter 8 is about.

I argue in later chapters that you need to make a conscious choice to restrict your calorie intake. This is a powerful choice. It will take a careful strategy, and you will have to be committed to this course of action.

Third, some folks say that you should "eat only when you are hungry." I think this piece of advice has been widely misunderstood to mean that "if you are hungry, then you should eat." In fact, nothing could be further from the truth!

I am predisposed towards being obese. My body sends me hunger signals all the time, even after a big meal. So, if I ate whenever I was hungry, I know that I would be morbidly obese by now.

Since I cannot trust the hunger signals I get from my body, I have to impose limits on what I eat and when I eat. I have to monitor my weight regularly. I have to know how much food I am allowed given my food "budget" (I do not count calories as such; rather, I am aware of what quantity and quality of food is right for me). Sticking to my food budget means that at least 20 times a day I have to choose not to eat, even when I am hungry.

Given my messed-up hunger signals, although being hungry is a *necessary* condition for eating, it is not a *sufficient* condition for eating. This is an important distinction, so, let me rephrase it. You should eat only *some* of the time that you are hungry, but not *all* of the time that you are hungry. You need to be hungry and unfulfilled more often than you would wish. Also, you should almost never eat if you are not hungry (a breakfast-related exception is discussed later).

Eating healthfully (both quantity and quality of food) regardless of your messed-up hunger signals is a conscious and powerful choice.

Fourth, I have an issue. I am hungry all the time. That feeling is alleviated only by eating large quantities of food. When I was younger, I did exactly that, and it made me fat. So, just over 30 years ago I made a conscious choice to not be fat any more. **I chose to be hungry all the time instead of being fat all the time.**

One of my friends read an early draft of this book and said that this last statement sounded terrible. He said that I had simply "substituted one misery for another." To the contrary, however, let me tell you that although being hungry all the time was hard work to begin with, once eating healthfully became a part of my routine, feeling hungry also became routine. That is, the hunger pains, although constant and gnawing, just faded into the background noise for the most part.

My hunger pains are contractions of muscles in my stomach, triggered by not having eaten as much as my brain wants me to eat. (The actual mechanism is very complex. See, for example, Garfield et al. [2015] and their references.) The pains come in cycles, and although I notice the peaks of those cycles, the pains settle down a little after a few minutes and then I can ignore them.

Feeling hungry all the time is an unpleasant feeling, but it is a better feeling to me than the feeling I had when I was fat all the time. I made a conscious, committed, powerful choice.

I will discuss different sorts of issues later. I don't know what your issues are, but I assume that whatever your particular issues are, they are something serious, or you would not be reading this book. So, whatever *your* issues are, you need to commit to addressing them.

Fifth, I think you need to stop looking for an outward crutch! For some folks, it is a weight loss group they belong to. For other folks, it is someone to talk to about their problems, or some sort of support group. Some folks cling to a bible, or prescription drugs, or some computer app for their smart-toy. Some folks pin their hopes on stomach surgery (which can certainly lead to weight loss, but can have some nasty side effects—discussed later). Other folks try crazy fad diet after crazy fad diet after crazy fad diet. All these things are crutches. None of them addresses the root cause of your problems.

The root cause of your problems is your unhealthy attitude and unhealthy behavior, which in turn are driven by your brain and its impulses. Ultimately, it is *you* who lifts your hand to your mouth and feeds your body too much food, or feeds your body junk food, or lights a cigarette, or chooses not to go out and get some exercise.

So, throw away the crutches and train yourself to be there for yourself, every day, from now on. This book is not a crutch, but a simple information source to help you set your course of action. You need to commit to being there for yourself when nobody else is. You are the only person who you can rely upon being there for you 24-7.

If you are religious, remember that God helps those who help themselves. Use your faith to enhance your empowerment. Religion is about looking inside of yourself. So, do some honest soul-searching, rather than praying for a miracle. Gluttony is a sin (because it hurts the body God gave you), and you must fight against it. Indeed, curbing bodily desires is a core part of most faith traditions, and this fits with, and reinforces, my disciplined approach.

You have to take ownership of the fact that you have issues. You have to be honest with yourself and with your friends and family. You have to make a conscious choice to recognize and take control of your issues.

Remember too that getting to a healthy weight is not a once-only event. You don't do it for a wedding, or for the summer. Rather, it is a way of life that you choose to live from now on. Otherwise, your weight will just yo-yo back to where it was, or worse.

For me, having weight issues is a bit like being an alcoholic, insofar as you will always be an alcoholic even when you have your drinking under control. Of course, alcoholics can stop drinking completely, but I cannot stop eating completely. So, it is different in that respect.

Let me add something else that many folks are afraid to say out loud for fear of persecution. If you choose to be fat and unhealthy by overeating and not exercising enough, and you choose to do nothing about it, then in the long run, looking after you will be a drain on the healthcare system, and upon your family.

It's not like someone smashed into your car when you were stopped at a red light. In that case, your healthcare costs are not caused by something that is your fault. If, however, you choose to eat unhealthy food in unhealthy quantities, then you are purposely choosing a course of action that will, when you are older, if not already, put a drain on the healthcare system. (See Chapter 10 for specific forecasts of the impact of your being fat on your life expectancy and on reductions in your healthy years of life remaining.)

This argument is especially true in a country with a national healthcare scheme, like the U.K., Canada, Australia, and N.Z. It may be unorthodox to say it, but in these countries I think it is downright unpatriotic and selfish to be fat or a smoker because you are asking everybody else to subsidize your unhealthy choices. Given national budget constraints in these countries, I would go so far as to say that if you are fat and unhealthy, then you are now, or soon will be, stealing social services from others who are in genuine need of it through no fault of their own but who cannot change their circumstances. In countries where the emphasis is more on a user-pays healthcare system (like the U.S.), then you are creating avoidable costs for yourself, and raising the general strain on the healthcare system.

I think all that is shameful. You need to take ownership of the problem, be honest about it, and do something about it so that you can hold your head up high. You may never have served in the military, but you can serve your country by committing to a healthy lifestyle now, reducing the future strain on the healthcare system, and freeing up healthcare resources for those who better need them.

Chapter 3

I Am Fat

I am fat. So, my goal is to lose weight, right? No, let me remind you that I said in the previous chapter that the goal is to get healthy, and by so doing, to attain a healthy weight.

As soon as you figure out that the aim is "to get healthy," and not "to lose weight," all those fad diets (low-carb, high-protein, caveperson, fruit, etc.) focused on weight loss fall by the wayside. For example, if a system or package is advertised with the slogan "Lose 10 pounds using our system," or something similar, then beware—that's the wrong goal and it is unlikely to work for you. Look somewhere else.

Similarly, if some company advertises with the slogan "Get slim for summer," then that's also a signal that this is unlikely to work for you. Getting healthy and staying healthy is about meeting long-term goals. Ideally, you want to see the slogan "Get healthy for life."

Indeed, anything that comes in a shake, or a plan, or a system, or a package, is not what you are looking for. How could that processed packaged food possibly be part of a long-term solution? It's just another homing pigeon for sale, as mentioned previously.

Ask yourself if you could eat those bars and drink those shakes for the rest of your life. If the answer is no, then it is a short-lived, faddish attempt at a fix, and anything short-lived is a crutch that will likely not put you on course for the long-term goal of being healthy.

Similarly, any diet involving the removal of familiar food groups or the imposition of unfamiliar food groups is a good sign that the proposed diet is a fad (see further discussion of fad diets in Chapter 6).

Let us now discuss concrete techniques for achieving the correct goal: getting healthy.

Chapter 4

Techniques for Getting Healthy

My combination of constant hunger, rapid weight gain, and slow weight loss, means that maintaining a healthy weight has been a constant battle, every day, for over 30 years now. There is definitely an obese person inside of me fighting to get out at every possible opportunity.

If you are reading this book, then you have issues. Perhaps it is the same hunger I have, perhaps it is the very slow metabolism that I have with the accompanying propensity to gain weight quickly and lose it slowly, perhaps it is depression, or sadness, or greed, or boredom, or guilt, or shame, or financial worries, or work stress, or family troubles, or loneliness, or post-traumatic stress disorder (PTSD), or something else. I assume that whatever your issues are, they are something serious.

The great majority of these issues are not your fault. They were caused by situations beyond your control and you had no choice in the matter. You cannot control the lousy hand that life already dealt you. You can, however, control what you do about it now.

In other words, if you see yourself as a victim of these lousy circumstances, then you will be a victim. If you choose to fight, however, then you can be a winner. For example, I am strongly genetically predisposed towards obesity, and I cannot change that, but I refuse to let that lousy situation determine my outcomes. I refuse to give in. It is a battle that I refuse to lose (I discuss this mental attitude further in Chapter 5).

You may be surprised to know that many of the issues I mentioned can be addressed, at least to some extent, by getting healthy. For example, depression is associated with obesity (Pratt and Brody, 2014), and exercise is reported to counter depression (HHL, 2013). Similarly, recent PTSD is associated with obesity (Pagoto et al., 2012), and exercise is reported to be beneficial at reducing PTSD symptoms (Hall et al., 2015).

Whatever your issue is, I think you need to aim at getting healthy. You need to eat less, eat more healthfully, and exercise more. It is that simple.

How do you go about eating less? Well, there are a number of tricks you may have to use to fool your body and brain into accepting fewer calories.

For example, when I first restricted my calorie intake, I would brush my teeth and then chew on a toothbrush between meals (about the house, but not in public). I found that brushing my teeth somehow drew a mental line under my eating, signaling that my meal was over. The action of chewing on something quite resilient was satisfying and kept my mind off eating. You might replace the toothbrush with chewing gum in public (which is acceptable in the U.S.), or chewing beeswax from a honeycomb (which has an interesting flavor).

Breakfast is my biggest meal of the day. I have to eat lunch at 11 A.M. because I simply cannot last any longer. I also have to eat a small supper to stave off hunger at night. You may be different.

In terms of addressing other issues, exercise can cheer you up (because of natural endorphins released into your blood stream), take your mind off bad things (because you need to concentrate when exercising), introduce you to other people (who are also exercising), and help to counter stress (because exercise is a stress release).

Are you eating because you're bored? If so, do something with yourself. Exercise should be the first thing on your list for all the reasons mentioned in the previous paragraph. It does not have to be running or lifting weights or anything very stressful to start with. Indeed, if you do pick something very stressful, "homeostasis" is likely to kick in and tell your brain to stop the exercise.

Homeostasis (pronounced "home-ee-oh-stay-sis") is when your brain reacts to external stimuli in an attempt to maintain the internal balance of your body. For example, your body sweats to cool you down when you get too hot, or shivers to warm you up when you get too cold, or slows your metabolism at the first hint of famine, to conserve calories. It is your body's self-preservation mechanism.

Homeostasis is what causes yo-yo dieting. That is, you lose some weight, but you gain it back again soon after because your body does not like shocks and tries to maintain its state.

So, you need to fool your body into accepting

gradual changes, rather than hitting your body with a sudden shock that it then tries to bounce back against. So, when picking an exercise routine to start with, pick a low-intensity exercise that you can sustain over time (HHL, 2013).

Homeostasis works the other way too. If I am at a healthy weight, and then I feast on the maximum food I can possibly consume for a week, gaining 25 pounds, my body will rebel, increasing my metabolic rate in an attempt to push my weight back to where it was.

Indeed, the only way you were able to gain as much weight as you have is by doing so gradually and fooling your body into accepting it. It took time and effort to do that. Now it is time to unwind the transformation. The unwinding will be slow too, though perhaps not quite as slow as the weight gain because the weight loss will be a deliberate act, whereas the weight gain was accidental. Any changes in food intake or changes in your exercise routine must be introduced gently enough to fool your body and brain into accepting them.

So, why not start by just going for a walk. You have to make it enough of a walk, however, that your body notices, not just a leisurely stroll, but not so much of a walk that homeostasis kicks in.

Work exercise into your daily routine. Walk to the store and bring two bags of groceries home instead of driving there once a week and bringing 10 bags home. Walk to work, or part way to work. Walk home, or part way home. It does not have to be every day; start off with every second day, or even once a week.

Do you love junk food (cookies, chips, chocolate bars, candy, soda, etc.)? If so, then do not keep a hoard of junk food in your house. It is way too tempting. Once a week, or better yet once a month, buy a small supply of treats, and do not restock until the month is up, even if you run out early. Treats are meant to be treats!

You are training your body, and your body needs a regular schedule. So, establish regular eating habits by having your meals at regular times. In addition to being simple common sense, there is some evidence that regular meal patterns may help with weight problems (Berg and Forslund, 2015).

You have to be sure to eat a good-sized breakfast. Different people need different-sized breakfasts. Some like a small breakfast and a big dinner; some the opposite. Just do not skip breakfast. It is called "breakfast" because you are breaking your overnight fast. Break-fast—get it?

If you skip breakfast, your body goes into "famine mode," or "fasting mode," and your brain will slow your metabolism down even further, multiply your feelings of hunger, and try to hold onto and store any calories you give it—in case the famine is a long-lasting one. This is another example of the homeostasis self-protection mechanism.

So, eat regular, good-sized meals. Not enough to fill you up, most likely, but enough to stop the famine mode kicking in. If you surprise or shock your body by missing meals or by having unexpected meals at unexpected times, you disrupt the training process. Either you end up eating more food than you need to or you shock your body into famine mode. So, the one exception to the "do not eat if you are not hungry" rule is that you should have a small breakfast even when you are not hungry, even just a piece of toast, so as not to upset your training schedule.

I think any meal may be viewed as breaking a fast, and the times between meals may be viewed as fasting. Some diet gurus condemn snacking between meals, but I think it depends upon the individual's needs. I certainly find that sometimes I need a small healthy snack between meals. Choose habits that work for you.

Individual calorie intakes vary dramatically from person to person. If eating your current calorie intake has gotten you fat, then once you reduce calories, you may find yourself eating much less than your spouse, your friends, even your little children (that's certainly been my experience!). Don't try to match their consumption. Thinking you were like other people may be part of what got you into trouble in the first place. Tell family and friends what you are doing so that they can revise their expectations of your intake.

If you get very hungry at night, then there are three things you can do. First, you can eat a small after-dinner supper just before you go to bed to help reduce the hunger pains. Second, when you are in bed, and get hunger pains, lie on your side and bring your knees up, but not all the way up to your chest. Third, you can use an extra blanket on the bed. Each of these techniques tends to counteract night-time hunger pains really well.

I cannot stress enough how important it is to use a small dinner plate and to take small portions of food (Berg and Forslund, 2015). Your eyes look at your food on your plate and send a message to your brain. You need to trick your brain into thinking there is more food there than there really is. So, even if everyone else in your family eats off of a big plate, take a small one for yourself. You can do this for breakfast, lunch, and dinner, and even when choosing the size of kids' lunchboxes. In addition, you can eat with a smaller spoon than other folks. So, use a teaspoon instead of a tablespoon or dessert spoon. It looks goofy, but I found that it really works.

Homeostasis is not just a short-term negative phenomenon. There are long-term homeostasis effects that can be positively beneficial. For example, when you lose a lot of weight, then as long as you are young enough, your stretched-out skin can recover and shrink back, and stretch marks can disappear.

If you gain weight when you are young but you wait until you are old to lose the weight, however, then you may need to plan on having some cosmetic surgery because your skin may not have enough elasticity of its own to bounce back and take up the slack. For example, I just read a story about an older woman who lost an extraordinary amount of weight, and the thing that surprised her the most was the great quantity of excess skin she had hanging off her body that needed to be surgically removed. She also had breast surgery for sagging breasts.

CHAPTER 4. TECHNIQUES FOR GETTING HEALTHY

I consider myself fortunate in that I was fat when I was younger and, although headed for major obesity problems, I chose to attain a healthy weight and maintain it. If it had happened the other way around, that is, if I had gotten fat as I got older and then lost the weight, I might have needed cosmetic surgery to remove loose skin flaps. In addition, if I had been fat when older, then that would have placed extra stress and strain on my aging cardio-vascular system and my aging joints. Nevertheless, even though I lost weight when I was younger, I still had stretch marks for several years.

Some folks have some sort of stomach surgery to restrict how much food they can eat. This is often very successful, because it mechanically restricts how much food you can fit into your stomach. Unfortunately, this sort of surgery is associated with a poor quality of life. You get stomach upsets, reflux, etc. You basically feel terrible.

Although the people I have known personally who have had stomach surgery did end up eating less food and losing weight, they were still making unhealthy food choices. That is, they were still eating junk food, just less of it because they would get physically sick if they ate too much. I think that their inability to make healthy food choices, both before and after the surgery, shows that they were, basically, the sort of people who could not make the committed choices I talk about in this book. Surgery was a last resort for them because it put a physical barrier (that is, reflux/vomiting) in place to stop them consuming too much food. The outcome would have been far superior for them if they could have made healthy food choices (both in terms of quality and quantity of their food) in the first place. Although they lost weight, and this improved their lives, they did not end up fully healthy. They did not meet the goal of achieving a healthy weight. I consider this a failure and additional evidence that weight loss is not the correct goal in the first place.

Some people are introverts; they don't need any sort of support from others. Some people are extroverts; they need people around them for support. For example, I read about a fat woman who lost 30 pounds. She said, however, that she was so fat to begin with that nobody noticed her weight loss. So, she felt discouraged about that and she gave up, and gained the weight back again. Clearly she did not have the inner resolve to do something just for herself.

Unfortunately, getting healthy is a very personal

affair. Nobody but you controls your food intake. Sure, you can go to others for information and hints, but success in attaining a healthy weight has to come from within. Quite frankly, if you are an extrovert or have emotional issues, then you may have difficulty losing weight.

You have to do this on your own. My opinion is that you should not join a gym, or some weight loss club, or buy into some weight loss program, or buy any expensive exercise gear. That's just setting yourself up for failure followed by failure, and it takes money out of your pocket too. At best, invest in a pair of very comfortable athletic shoes.

Only if you are an extreme and incurable extrovert should you join any sort of weight loss group. As I said earlier, I think support groups are a crutch that does not address the root problem—which is *you* and *your attitude.* I view these support groups as a costly diversion of time away from working on your issues and the healing or addressing of them from within.

In fact, I fear that sometimes support networks could be part of what got you into trouble in the first place. Other people invite you to go to dinner with them, or out drinking, or they eat big meals with you (relative to what would be healthy for you). They are part of your support network to stay fat! If you want success, it has to come from within. You may have to socialize less to be able to work on your own issues; you may even be labelled anti-social.

The bottom line is that you have to take ownership of your issues, admit that you are fat, and unhealthy, and that it is your fault and nobody else's. Maybe life dealt you a lousy hand, but it is you, and it has always been you, who is in control of your outcomes. So, commit to making a change. Make your powerful choice to not put up with being fat any longer and to start the slow process towards getting healthy.

Chapter 5

Psychology

I have a slim and inexpensive book called *The Dirty Dozen* sitting on my bookshelf. At least once a year, I take it off the shelf and reread it. It is written by Sergeant Major (Ret.) Lawrence A. Jordan. Jordan served a 24-year Special Operations career with the U.S. Army Rangers and Special Forces. His book (Jordan, 2002) is about dirty fighting techniques, and Chapter 2, "The Winning Mind," is about mental preparation for life-or-death, hand-to-hand combat in self-defense. Jordan argues that in combat you must adopt the mental attitude that you simply "refuse to lose."

I recommend "The Winning Mind" chapter of

Sergeant Major Jordan's book because you too are facing a life-or-death fight. Sure enough, nobody is pointing a gun at you or charging at you with a machete. There is no *immediate* threat of death or dismemberment, but the threat is just as real nevertheless (see the terrible statistics on loss of years of life in Chapter 10). So, I strongly recommend that you read this particular chapter in Jordan's book. I think you will find more there for you than you are expecting.

I mentioned guilt and depression previously. Those are not my issues. I think, however, that eating yourself to death and failing to exercise is like some kind of long-run suicide, and that choosing to be obese is, for some people, a "cry for help" akin to the cry for help often attributed to people who attempt suicide.

When you choose to be fat and unhealthy, you stand out as someone who is in need of help and who is preparing themselves for and accelerating their own death. You may think that this sounds extreme, but if you are choosing to preside over this slow-moving train wreck, what am I supposed to think? How do you think this looks from the outside?

The bottom line is that there is one and only one

person who is going to help you with this problem. Go look in the mirror to see who that person is.

Stop crying for help; it is not coming. Accept now that getting healthy is something you have to do yourself. Take ownership of your health issues. Make your committed choice now to get healthy. Refuse to lose!

Chapter 6

Food and Health

It is time to be honest with yourself and others. Are you under the impression that you do not eat too much? If so, then it is time to think again. If you are fat now, then you have been putting too many calories into your body relative to the calories you have been burning. It is simple body arithmetic.

Look at what you are eating. Look at the quantity and the quality of your food. Most people, regardless of education, know the difference between healthy food and unhealthy food. Is there junk food in your diet? Do you eat deep-fried food? Do you eat out at restaurants more than once a week? (Restaurant food is often calorie-dense.) Alcohol is very caloric. Do you drink alcohol more than once a week? Too many calories is part of what got you into this mess. Healthy people eat and drink only in moderation. You need to be more like them. So, eat less, eat more healthfully, and exercise more.

Ask yourself also whether you have passed your unhealthy behavior on to members of your family, either through your genes (nature), or through your actions (nurture). In either case, the outcome is the same and needs to be addressed.

I said that I think most people know the difference between healthy and unhealthy food. Wholemeal bread is healthy; white bread is not. Water is healthy; sweetened soda (either natural or artificial sweetener) is not healthy. An orange is healthy; orange-flavored candy is not. Raw nuts are healthy; roasted nuts are not.

Unfortunately, some food masquerades as healthy when it is not. For example, many oat-based granola/muesli bars are little more than candy. Many "healthy" breakfast cereals with healthy names are full of fat, sugar, and fake flavorings (it's on the label!). Some dried fruit snacks made from fruit juice are really just candy. Similarly, a glass of orange juice is nowhere near as healthy as an orange, and sweetened yogurt is nowhere near as healthy as natural unsweetened yogurt.

The more processing involved in your food, the less healthy the outcome. In a similar vein, the longer the list of ingredients on the packet of your grocery item, the less healthy the contents. Read the labels. Three ingredients is likely healthy, but 30 ingredients is a chemistry experiment!

Note that food that says "99 percent fat free" is often full of sugar, and food that says "low GI" or "low sugar" is often high in fat. You don't have to eat like a caveperson, but at the same time, you should not be eating as if you are on the last stage of a mission to Mars (and all you have left is heavily processed food).

I have mentioned fad diets several times already. Let me now explain clearly something about fad diets that I have never heard anyone say. There exist fad diets that emphasize some healthy food groups, while simultaneously demonizing other food groups. Perhaps they demonize dairy, or grains, or carbohydrates, or red meat, or fish, or beans, or something else. Well, if you currently have *really terrible* eating habits, then one of these fad diets may be better for you than the habits you currently follow. So, following the fad diet may be an improvement over the terrible eating habits you have now, and the fad diet could be a step in the direction of reaching your goal of getting healthy. Let me explain, however, why no fad diet can get you all the way to your goal of getting healthy.

In almost all cases, you are not unhealthy because of grains, or dairy, or carbohydrates, or red meat, or fish, or beans, or any sensible food group. Rather, you are unhealthy because either the quantity of food you have been eating is unhealthy (that is, too many calories), or the quality of food you have been eating is unhealthy (for example, too much junk food, or alcohol, or candy), or you have not been getting enough healthy exercise, or, most likely, because of some combination of all three of these issues.

A healthy diet is one that includes all things in moderation. For example, it's fine to have some junk food or candy as a treat, or to drink alcohol (if you are not pregnant), but it has to be in moderation. See, for example, the Harvard School of Public Health's recent Healthy Eating Pyramid (HSPH, 2012). Note that Harvard's food pyramid fixes fundamental flaws in the USDA's outdated Food Pyramid that was originally introduced back in 1992 (see HSPH [2012]).

Healthy people do not exclude whole food groups for health reasons. (Of course, some people do exclude a food group for religious or ethical reasons.) Rather, healthy people eat a varied diet, with moderation in all things. If you listen to the public media, however, you will hear people shouting out the benefits of this or that fad diet that demonizes some food group(s). Just because they are loud, does not make them right!

Let me give you an analogy. If I am in San Francisco, and my goal is to get to Boston, but the only flight leaving is going to Chicago, in-between, then sure enough, getting on that flight gets me closer to my goal; but hey, I am still not in Boston, and I still need to take more action to reach my goal! Similarly, if I have a terrible diet, and I switch over to the fad diet that includes lots of healthy fruit and vegetables, but demonizes grains and dairy, say, then sure enough, I will likely feel healthier than I did; but hey, that's still not a healthy diet, and I will still have to include the healthy food groups, in moderation, along with exercise, also in moderation, to get to my goal.

So, of course the fad diet promoters can find people (especially those with previously *terrible* eating habits) who will give testimonials to say that they have benefited from the fad diet, but that does not make the fad diet healthy, or part of a long-term plan to get healthy. If you treat the fad diet as a stepping stone on the way to a healthy diet, then that is fine, but you need to recognize that the fad diet is not your final destination.

(As an aside, I think that some folks like the strict rules associated with fad diets because their lives/diets are currently out of control and they crave structure. If you need structure, then look for it in reduced calorie intake, regular timing of your meals, regular exercise, high-quality food, etc. Do not look for it in food group restrictions that, upon closer examination, are unhealthy.)

There are, of course, folks with diseases who will benefit from an exclusionary diet. For example, roughly 1 percent of people in most nations have celiac/coeliac disease (pronounced "see-lee-ack")(Fasano et al., 2015; Green et al., 2015). People with this disease have improved health outcomes by excluding foods containing gluten. Another 3–6 percent of people have nonceliac gluten sensitivity (NCGS).[1]

Recent evidence questions, however, whether

---

[1]Figure 1 of Fasano et al. (2015) provides a clear classification of gluten-related disorders, including celiac dis-

gluten is even what people with NCGS are react-
ing to, because removing some specialized types of
carbohydrates (called FODMAPs) from their diets
appears to alleviate their symptoms (Biesiekierski
et al., 2013; Vanga and Leffler, 2013). However,
these FODMAPs occur in such a low dose in gluten-
containing grains that it is not obvious that these
are the issue either (Fasano et al., 2015). Thus, the
exact nature of NCGS is still very much open to
debate.

The bottom line is, therefore, that for something like 93–99 percent of the population, excluding gluten from the diet without formal medical
testing may be a naive decision partly driven by
inappropriate fad diets (Fasano et al., 2015). By all
means do what works for you, but educate yourself
first and seek professional advice where appropri-
ate.

I ignore fads, and I impose structure based on a
common sense approach to healthy eating. For example, I have found that sticking to a habit helps
me. So, I eat pretty much the same breakfast every
day, the same lunch every day, and then a healthy
dinner that varies a lot from day to day. Having

---

ease, wheat allergy, and NCGS. The authors also distinguish
clearly between food sensitivity and food intolerance.

chosen the correct size for my meals, eating the same breakfast and lunch every day is then a type of self-imposed portion control (see the scientific discussion of portion control in Berg and Forslund [2015]).

For lunches at work, at the beginning of the week I buy a bunch of bananas and a loaf of wholegrain bread (no preservatives). I keep the bread in the freezer at home, and I take out three slices each morning to take to the office in a bag. I buy the healthiest peanut butter I can stomach (usually just peanuts and minimal salt). I keep the bananas and peanut butter at work. Then each day for lunch I have two bananas and three slices of wholegrain bread with peanut butter, usually eaten at my desk, accompanied by a glass of water. That daily lunch picks off several items on the Harvard School of Public Health's Healthy Eating Pyramid (HSPH, 2012). It is cheap, fast, easy, healthy, and sustaining. Find something similarly healthy that suits your palate.

When invited to work-related, non-dinner events with food and drink, I rarely eat anything because it is usually unhealthy food, and I drink only water. I have only a limited number of calories to spend on my food budget, and unhealthy food is simply not worth the calories. By sticking to those habits, I know that I am not varying much in my consumption. I will not slowly and accidentally start consuming too much food again. At work-related dinners, I usually eat sparingly.

Speaking of eating dinners, I have to tell you to stop wolfing down your food. I once sat down to dinner with an obese friend of mine. We talked as I slowly ate my food. She moved her food around on the plate barely touching it. When I was nearly done, her plate was still full. I thought maybe she did not like her food. Two minutes later, when I was done, however, I looked up and her plate was clean. She had finished before me, eating her entire dinner in one-tenth the time it took me to eat the same quantity!

Like my friend, I too have the ability to wolf down my food; it helped keep me fat when I was younger. When you eat slowly, however, you make a healthy quantity of food last much longer. You may also be giving your body more time for a network of inter-related hormonal signals to take effect, signaling that you have eaten enough (HMHL, 2010). Eating slowly is also better for your digestion and for your body's ability to extract nutrients from your food. So, eat more slowly, starting today.

You need to savor your food more, both because you will be getting less of it in the future and because it is a healthy choice.

Some weight loss advisors recommend drinking lots of water to stave off hunger pains. Sure enough, drinking water can briefly bring a feeling of fullness, or at least a feeling of heaviness in your belly.

Drinking lots of water can, however, put a strain on your kidneys. Drinking lots of water also dilutes your stomach acids, and this can bring on indigestion. Diluted stomach acid is also less likely to kill off bacteria in food, so this increases your risk of food poisoning, or at least getting sick from your food. Finally, drinking lots of water sends you off to the bathroom all the time, including in the middle of the night.

Some folks recommend eight glasses of water a day. That's fine if you live in the U.S., with central heating in the winter and air conditioning in the summer. If you live in a cold house in N.Z., however, with no central heating and no air conditioning, then eight glasses of water may be way too much. For example, one of the first things I noticed when moving from N.Z. to the U.S., was that I had to almost immediately double my water intake. Perhaps this heating/cooling effect is one reason why sodas became so popular in the U.S.

Note too that although eight glasses of water a day may make sense for a large person, it might not make sense for a smaller person.

So, drink plenty of water, even a little more than usual, but not so much that you feel like you are drowning in it or running to the bathroom all the time.

Watch out also for media-driven fads. For example, the media might report that red wine is healthy because the French have fewer health issues than Americans. My personal opinion is that this is mostly bogus. I spent a total of three months living in France, and the French are healthier than the Americans because of their attitude towards the living of life. The French are relaxed about many things that Americans are uptight about; it is part of their culture. Don't assume that you can adopt their diet and reap the benefits if you don't adopt their lifestyle!

Speaking of lifestyles, I watched a television show once where a group of people were judging some food. A very fit-looking man declared the food to be "way too salty." A fat woman declared that the fit man was dead wrong, and that the food was not salty at all. They argued back and forth about what each thought was patently obvious— but each missed what was obvious to me. Namely, that the fit man usually ate a healthy diet and the food placed in front of him on the show had too much salt relative to his normal healthy diet. The fat woman, however, usually ate an unhealthy diet and so the food seemed normally salted to her. She had an oversalted palate.

Every time I eat out at a restaurant nowadays I am struck by how very salty and fatty the food is. I have found this in N.Z., the U.K., the U.S., and even France. If you eat out at restaurants and do *not* think the food is salty, then you likely have an oversalted palate, but you might not know it.

I have a friend who comes to visit on occasion. We do not keep a salt shaker on the dining room table. So, he always goes and gets some salt from our kitchen and sprinkles it on his already correctly salted food. He has an oversalted palate because he has trained his palate to accept that. He also has high blood pressure (which often goes hand in hand with a high salt intake). If you keep salt shakers on the dining room table, then my guess is that you likely have an oversalted palate—unless you routinely use no salt in the preparation of your food.

Why is restaurant food so over salted? It is

because it is meant to be a treat, and treats often have high salt, or high fat, or high sugar, or many calories, or a combination of some or all of these.

When you eat out frequently at restaurants, you are rewarding yourself with constant treats, but not as a reward for anything meaningful. How can you ever have a treat, or enjoy anything as a treat, if you have treats all the time? It is like having Christmas every day. How is anything special any more if you cannot delay some of that gratification and take control of your life?

I think you need to develop the capacity to enjoy less of something. Less is more! You won't get this outcome by overconsuming treats. For example, when I have a slice of pizza nowadays, I really enjoy it. When I go to a restaurant, I am very particular about my choice of restaurant and my choice of food because maybe I only get to go once every two or three months. It is a real treat for me. Even so, I still tend to order smaller portions than most people when I do go to a restaurant, because of the importance of choosing small portions (Berg and Forslund, 2015).

Eating restaurant food or takeout food has another bad side effect. If children (and perhaps you) are given the opportunity to eat restaurant food and takeout food too often, then many times they get what they want without having to challenge their palates. That is, the children (and you) are following the path of least resistance. You should instead be trying new vegetables and healthy cooking, not taking the easy way out where you just point at what you want and pay for it. If children's palates are not challenged, you may be setting them up for unhealthy choices in the future.

I remember switching from full-fat milk to low-fat milk 30 years ago. After a few months, if I tried full-fat milk it just tasted like a creamy custard treat. It does not take long to retrain the palate; less than a year in that case.

As a professor, I advise students who are going out to interview for jobs. They often seem surprised that I know they are smokers, because they simply cannot smell it any more. I tell them to quit or get a patch or something similar because some employers, especially white-collar employers, would never knowingly hire a smoker.

The good thing about all this is that it is easy to diagnose, and easy to fix. If you smoke, and don't think you smell of smoke, then you are anosmic to it (anosmia is to noses, what blindness is to eyes). If you don't think restaurant food is salty, then you have an oversalted palate for sure.

Quit smoking and stop adding any salt to your food. Reduce restaurant visits to no more than once or twice per month. If you think this goal is laughingly unrealistic, then I urge you to reconsider. Restaurant food is treat food! Eating it often is helping to make you fat. If you want to get healthy, you have to change your lifestyle. Do it gradually, so as not to shock your body.

Of course, you should note that some people with fast metabolisms or mild hunger signals can eat lots of restaurant food without getting fat. They are, however, still unhealthy internally because of their unhealthy food choices. This is yet another reminder that weight loss is not the goal.

You might ask what does salt or smoking have to do with losing weight. Let me remind you that the goal is not losing weight (attaining that goal tends to fail), but rather the goal is getting healthy and thereby attaining a healthy weight. High salt intake and smoking are not healthy and are not part of attaining a healthy weight.

As an aside, let me tell you a short story about smoking. When I finished my PhD at MIT, I bought myself a mountain bike in Boston as a graduation present. When I first lived in central London, I would go out riding my bike on Sunday mornings (lots of folks are unaware that London closes off a whole bunch of roads to cars on Sunday mornings, so you can walk or cycle unmolested all the way from Kensington Palace to Trafalgar Square if you wish).

One problem with cycling in London, however, is that the air quality is very poor, even on a Sunday morning. So, like many London cyclists, I bought a carbon-filtered breathing mask and wore it while cycling. (Many other cyclists also wear a bandana over their breathing mask for an extra layer of protection.) Whenever I stopped to take a drink from my water bottle, I would remove the mask and immediately notice the dirty air, like a slap in the face. So, the mask was clearly very good at keeping the air pollutants out.

If I cycled past smokers, however, I could always smell their cigarette smoke even with my mask on. The particles of cigarette smoke were so fine, I think, that they went right through the filters in my mask. I have always assumed that the very fine nature of the cigarette smoke particles is what allows them to embed themselves in your lungs, and is one of the reasons smoking damages your body and can give you lung cancer, among other ailments.

I may be mistaken, but nevertheless it serves as a reminder of the dangers of smoking.

Speaking of damage to your body, note that if you have been feeding yourself an inappropriate quantity, and an inappropriate quality, of food for years, then you may have done some damage to your digestive system. Even when you reach a healthy weight, you may find that you still have digestive issues and bowel health issues. So, I strongly recommend a probiotic pill morning and evening to help sort you out. These pills contain the same organisms that appear in good yogurt, and they are often recommended after a course of antibiotics. In theory, you take them for a month and then everything is fine. In practice, however, you may find that you take them for much longer.

Similarly, if you have been eating unhealthy food in great quantity, you may actually be suffering from malnutrition. Yes, malnutrition is common among adults even in a first-world country like the U.S., and is even more common among the obese and overweight (Agarwal et al., 2015) and among older adults (Pereira et al., 2015). So, you might wish to add a multivitamin pill to your daily routine, at least until you include a reasonable number of healthy foods in your diet.

There is evidence, however, both that multivitamins added to an already healthy diet can increase cancer risks (Martínez et al., 2012) and that many users take multivitamins based on fad-like motivations (Martínez et al., 2012). Alternative, but not contrary, advice is that you should continue with your multivitamin, but avoid heavily fortified foods that might lead to overdosing on folic acid (HSPH, 2015). You get to choose, but do be aware that once your diet is healthy, multivitamins are not obviously necessary. Do be careful in choosing a multivitamin in the first place, because there can be side effects like constipation, etc. So, take some informed advice, most likely from a good doctor or dietician, before choosing what, if any, vitamin to take.

Do you drink sodas? The kind with sugar or the kind with fake sugar? Neither is healthy. When U.S. academics come to work at my N.Z. university, they often suck down sodas like they think they contain the antidote. The empty soda cans pile up in their office and they stand out as clearly coming from a different culture. There has been some sort of U.S. obsession with drinking soda instead of water, perhaps largely driven by advertising campaigns in the U.S. That advertising blitz never happened in N.Z., so U.S. visitors to N.Z. seem odd and unhealthy when they behave in that way.

Of course, it is difficult to see it as odd if you live in the U.S. and you are surrounded by like-minded, soda-drinking people. To an outsider, however, it looks as if U.S. folks who are drinking lots of sodas are gullible, having fallen prey to marketing from big soda companies. Why would you pay anything for unhealthy sweetened carbonated water?

As of 2015, U.S. soda sales have been dropping every year for 10 years (Esterl, 2015), with Diet Coke sales falling for eight consecutive years (Kell, 2015). That's a great trend, but it is not enough. If you are drinking soda, the only ingredients should be water and carbon dioxide. Maybe a hint of citrus or something similar is alright, but anything beyond that is unhealthy. So, give up the unhealthy sodas. Your palate will quickly retrain to the new, healthier, soda, or just plain water.

I saw an alarming statistic released in early 2015. For the first time since the Department of Commerce started recording data in 1992, Americans spent more money on restaurant food and bars than they spent buying groceries (Jamrisko, 2015). That does not necessarily mean that they ate out more frequently than in, because restaurant food is more expensive than supermarket food, but it does betray the alarming effort required to support the obesity epidemic.

I saw a television series once where each week a healthy person and a fat person swapped food intakes for a week. The healthy person was always amazed at how long it took to consume the food intake of the fat person. They would sit there shoveling it down, and have reactions like "Oh God, not more. How the hell am I going to eat this?" and after eating it, they would have a reaction like "Oh God, I feel so stuffed I think I am going to vomit." In contrast, the fat person would gobble the healthy person's food in a minute and bemoan the small quantity, wondering how they could possibly make it through the rest of the day on so little food. At the end of the show, the producer would fill two wide vertical glass tubes with the food usually eaten by each person in a week, so that the differences in both quality and quantity were clearly visible. The contrast in quantity and color was amazing. There were lots of dull processed greys and browns in the fat person's overstuffed glass tube, and a colorful rainbow of fruit and vegetables in the healthy person's under-stuffed glass tube.

Speaking of groceries, I would like to suggest that the next time you are in the supermarket, you find a fit/healthy looking person in the store and follow them around and see what they buy. Carry your shopping list in one hand and a basket in the other and keep looking at the list and putting things in your basket so that nobody gets suspicious. Then compare what they buy with what you usually buy. My guess is that they will not be buying sugary sodas, high-sugar foods, or high-fat foods. They will likely spend quite a bit of time in the produce section, and they will likely be stopping to read labels. If they do buy treats, they will likely be buying only a small quantity of them. So, if you want to be more like them, then take a leaf out of their book and shop more like them.

If you are going to tilt your diet towards healthier food, then fewer restaurant visits are essential. It goes without saying that if you are eating less restaurant food, then you are eating more food at home. It takes time and effort to plan healthy meals. It also takes time and effort to shop for them. When you go to the supermarket (or wherever you buy your food), you need to have allowed yourself plenty of time to make healthy choices.

Maybe you were going to buy orange juice, but oranges are on sale today. Maybe you were going to buy beef, but there are no lean (that is, low-fat) cuts, and you have to look at fish instead. Maybe you need to spend some time in the cereal aisle looking for a breakfast cereal that is lower in sugar than your usual choice (for example, regular oatmeal/porridge versus processed sugar-coated wheat flakes). It takes time to make healthy choices in the market.

It does not help that the owners of the supermarket often place the less healthy items within easy reach, while placing the healthy items on the very bottom shelf, or in otherwise less obvious places. The market can charge more, or charge a higher markup, for the more processed food because peoples' modern palates like that food more (which in turn is one reason why the manufacturers processed it more in the first place).

The ideal meal is one that is delicious, healthy, cheap, easy to make (that is, very little skill is needed), and quick to make (that is, it uses little time to prepare and/or little time to cook). If you try to make a list of ideal dinner meals that meet all these criteria, however, you will likely find that the list is very short. It's like looking for the ideal mate, or the ideal house, or the ideal outfit. You are likely going to have to make a compromise somewhere.

My experience is that if you want healthy food,

the compromise is in the "easy to make" or "quick to make" criteria. Maybe it is easy to make, but you have to make it in a slow cooker, or maybe it cooks very quickly, but the preparation time is lengthy (planning for it, shopping for it, and physically standing over it in the kitchen at home while you make it). Again, it comes down to time and effort. It takes time and effort to prepare healthy food.

Note too that you might spend considerable time and effort planning for, shopping for, and then preparing a healthy meal, only to see it eaten in a short space of time. If this is your role in the household, it can seem a little disheartening to do this every day and see the fruits of your labor consumed so quickly, and perhaps with little thanks. It helps to remember that good health takes time and effort, and that everything you do pays off eventually.

If you look back to the time before WWII, most women worked in the home, and most men were the breadwinners. So, women had plenty of time to plan, shop, prepare, cook, and present healthy meals. During WWII, however, men were called upon in great numbers to serve overseas. So, women took men's places in factories and on farms to support the war effort and to maintain production on the home front. Women proved they had many of the same skills as men, and women entered the workforce in increasing numbers after WWII. Over the 70 years since WWII, the proportion of women in the U.S. labor force increased steadily from roughly 30 percent to roughly 60 percent (BLS, 2014). Simultaneously, the proportion of men in the labor force fell steadily from about 85 percent to about 70 percent (BLS, 2014).

On top of this, our increasing adoption of technology, especially since about 1980, has added stress to our lives instead of reducing stress. For example, when I was a child, various futurologists were forecasting that technology would reduce the length of the work week. The forecast was that by the year 2000, many of us would be working from home with dramatically increased leisure time. In practice, however, we are working more hours than ever, and we are constantly interrupted by phone calls, text alerts, emails, etc. This techno-stress gives us less leisure time, not more.

The bottom line is that now, more than at any prior time in history, there is less likely to be someone at home (male or female) who does not work outside the home. So, this presents an extra challenge when it comes to the time-consuming task of planning, shopping, preparing, and presenting healthy meals at home.

On top of this, if you are fat and living alone, cooking for one presents its own unique challenges. It can be difficult to judge correct portion sizes, and there is nobody there to give you a second opinion. So, this makes it all the more important that you educate yourself and are there for yourself 24-7.

(As an aside, looking back over the last 50+ years, I cannot help but notice that in photographs from the 1950s, 1960s, and even the 1970s, almost everyone looks very slim relative to the people of today. However, it is not that they are slim, it is that we are fat!)

Let me now tell some stories to make some points about issues with food.

My wife told me that when she was young she peered into the window of a neighbor's house. The man who lived there was fat. He was seated at his dining room table, alone, in front of a big chocolate cake. You can imagine almost any background story to that event, but none of them is a healthy story. The guy obviously had issues.

Here is another story. We were in Davis, California to visit relatives, and we went into a small restaurant to get some dinner. The food was of low quality, but the restaurant was near our hotel and we were tired after 25+ hours of planes and airports, etc. The biggest man I have ever seen in person came in and sat at the table next to us with his friend. He proceeded to order the largest meal I have ever seen anyone consume. It was served to him on the largest plates I have ever seen in a restaurant. I believe that there was, basically, no way he could maintain his weight at that high level without eating in bulk. I heard him declare to the waitress that it was his birthday. I could not help but wonder how many more he had left. It was really quite sad to see.

As mentioned previously, people who behave this way are, for whatever reason, committing a slow suicide. They are literally eating themselves to death. Unlike someone who surprises you by jumping off a tall building, you can see the suicide in progress over a period of years. It is a pitifully slow train wreck.

On a different note, there is a crime in the financial markets known as an "affinity fraud" (SEC, 2012). This is a crime that is perpetrated by a fraudster upon people in some group with which the fraudster has an affinity (that is, something in common). Oftentimes the fraudsters target people belonging to the same religious group, or belonging to the same ethnic group, or working in the same industry, or former veterans of the same military unit, etc. Sometimes even their affinity is faked (SEC, 2012).

If you are fat and unhealthy, then it would not surprise me to find that you spend a lot of time in the company of other people who are fat and unhealthy. Perhaps it is your friends, or your family, or a social group, or a religious group, or an ethnic group, or some other group with which you have an affinity. If you are embedded in some group of people that is reinforcing your unhealthy lifestyle, then it is time for you to be a leader, not a follower. Leaders turn their backs on followers; that is what followers deserve! You need to declare to your peers that you are sick and tired of being fat and unhealthy and that you are committed to making a change.

Have you ever noticed that one of the conditions of parole for criminals is that they not associate with other criminals? This is for fear that they will fall back into their old habits. Well, you likely do not want to be choosing new friends, but you may need to be a leader among them. Declare to them that you are not going to act like that any more.

Tell them you are going for a walk tomorrow and ask if they would like to join you.

Note that your brain and body need healthy food and proper hydration to function properly. Over the years, I have definitely noticed a very strong relationship between what I eat and how I perform on high-level mental or physical tasks. For example, as a part of my job, I need to perform in a university classroom for one or two hours at a time in front of large audiences (sometimes more than 500 persons). These performances typically involve demonstrations and explanations of deeply complicated mathematical concepts or high-level theoretical arguments, and I have to interact with the audience and think on my feet. There is no way I could do this on a diet of junk food and soda.

On a related note, I firmly believe that students with poor diets are undermining their ability to learn and perform, and thereby failing to reach their potential at college. I view this as a shameful waste of human health and opportunity, because once those years and those door-opening opportunities are gone, they cannot be easily found again.

Finally, pregnancy and breastfeeding deserve a special note here. I was a strong supporter of my wife when she was nursing our children, and

I have strong views on the benefits of breastfeeding. I recognize, however, that many folks have equally strong and opposing views. I know also that not all women are able to breastfeed—including many who very much want to do so. I recognize also that I am a male academic whose specialty is not in medicine. Given those acknowledgements, I will point at the American Academy of Pediatrics (AAP) Policy Statement recommendations and at recent published medical research in top journals. I am not so much giving my views on the topic, as I am summarizing advice from the experts in the area. These views, in my opinion, do not get much airplay both because they are often buried where the layperson won't see them, and because they are currently unpopular. You can choose to ignore what I present here, but at least you will be making an informed decision, not an uninformed one.

Most women who get pregnant gain an extra 25 pounds or more in addition to the weight of the baby. When your baby nurses, however, he or she takes high-energy milk out of your system. This activity, left to run its natural course, should, in theory, consume the extra weight you gained, until your weight returns slowly roughly to where it was before the baby was conceived.

Scientific evidence that breastfeeding promotes weight loss during the first two years after birth is mixed, but the most carefully executed studies support the expected relationship (Neville et al., 2014). In addition, looking at six years after birth, there is strong evidence of greater weight loss in obese mothers who breastfed their child following common recommendations, compared with obese mothers who did not breastfeed their child (Sharma et al., 2014).

What are the "common recommendations" just mentioned? Sharma et al., (2014) draw upon the AAP Policy Statement recommendation (Gartner et al., 2005), but use a slightly more conservative guideline that mothers should breastfeed exclusively for at least four months, with continued breastfeeding until at least the age of 12 months.

In fact, the AAP Policy Statement recommendation (Gartner et al., 2005) suggests that **exclusive breastfeeding for roughly six months is sufficient for optimal growth and development and that continued breastfeeding should take place until at least 12 months of age, and after that for as long as mutually desired by mother and child** (Gartner et al., 2005, p. 499). A revised AAP policy statement reaffirms more clearly the six-month exclusive breastfeeding recommendation without changing the other recommendations (Eidelman and Schanler, 2012). These AAP documents are easy to read, and packed full of useful information; I strongly recommend them.

Of course, in developed countries like the U.K. and the U.S., it is common for mothers to breastfeed for only the first six months or even less (Sugarman and Kendall-Tackett, 1995; Parkin, D.M., 2011; Foterek et al., 2014). Some U.S. mothers do, however, nurse for an extended period (Sugarman and Kendall-Tackett, 1995).

In addition to probable weight loss benefits for the mother, there is probable evidence that breastfeeding for more than one year reduces the likelihood of subsequent breast cancer (Parkin, 2011; Saslow, 2013) and ovarian cancer (Parkin et al., 2011; Su et al., 2013) in the mother, and that being breastfed reduces the likelihood of subsequent weight gain in the child (WCRF/AICR, 2007). Breastfeeding also presents dozens of other benefits for mother and child not mentioned here (Gartner et al., 2005; Eidelman and Schanler, 2012).

I know from personal family experience that breastfeeding is time-consuming hard work, and requires dedicated commitment. I also understand that for working mothers, in particular, breastfeeding longer than six months can be a big challenge. Pumping and storing your milk at work may be one option for working mothers, and a good business case can be made for doing this (Eidelman and Schanler, 2012), but I do not underestimate the practical difficulties of doing so.

There are also community benefits from breastfeeding. If you breastfeed as long as possible, you are helping to reduce the future strain on the healthcare system for yourself and your future grown-up child (Gartner et al., 2005; Eidelman and Schanler, 2012).

Breastfeeding is a natural, normal, healthy path to a healthy life for you and your child. Like many parts of a healthy life, it is hard work, requiring dedicated commitment. If you need breastfeeding information or support, contact your local Le Leche League (you can look them up on the Internet to find the nearest branch).

Chapter 7

It's Not Me; It's My Metabolism

It's not me; it's my metabolism.

No. Don't blame your metabolism. It is not your metabolism, it is you. It has always been you. I was in your shoes and in your head. I did not change the course of my life until I took ownership of my issues. So, be honest with yourself, starting right now.

Sure enough, your metabolism may be slow (so, you burn fewer calories than other folks doing the same work), but that's no excuse. That's just shifting the blame. Nobody has tied you down to force-feed you. It is *your* brain lifting *your* arm to put *your* choice of food (quantity and quality) into *your* mouth. It is *your* brain not taking *your* body out for exercise. There is nothing else and nobody else to blame.

Blaming your metabolism is like saying the availability of easy credit is to blame for overspending on your credit cards. Do not blame other enablers; not your spouse, not your family, not your friends, not the social situations you find yourself in, and certainly not your metabolism. Be honest!

In my experience, obesity has a lot to do with being dishonest in one way or another. You eat that extra piece of food even though you know your body does not need it; that's dishonest. You tell other people you are trying to lose the weight, but you have not been trying very hard to adopt a healthy lifestyle. You were never committed fully to it. You were looking for easy ways out. You kept on lifting your hand to your mouth too often and not taking the exercise you needed. That was dishonest. You lied to other people about it and you lied to yourself.

My experience is that many fat people are also uncomfortable eating what they want to eat in front of other people. This was true of me when I was overweight and is still true of me to some degree as some sort of holdover issue. I think there is an embarrassment associated with eating in public, and that this is related to dishonesty regarding what and how much you usually eat.

So, stop it right now. Admit that "I am fat and I am sick and tired of it." Tell your friends and family exactly that. Say it out loud. Accept it, embrace your acceptance of it, and commit to making the choices that healthy people make. It is hard work, but all the effort you currently put into eating, being dishonest with others and yourself, and not exercising can be redirected towards getting healthy instead.

Sometimes I see statements from doctors in the popular press to the effect that the body mass index (BMI) is not a meaningful measure of body fat for some racial groups. Doctors state that people from these racial groups should not pay attention to their BMI because people from these groups are naturally "big" or "heavy" or something similar, and that this predisposition biases the numbers.

I find these BMI-related statements to be complete hogwash. I believe that this is yet another case of doctors not wanting to tell people that "attaining a healthy weight is within your control, but it will take hard work." Doctors freely tell cancer patients that their chemotherapy will be hard on them, so why not tell obesity patients that the powerful choices they need to make will be hard too? I think doctors assume that these folks will not have the intestinal fortitude to adopt a healthy lifestyle, and so they write them off as not worthy of their time. It may be bordering on racism in this case. This medical advice then provides yet another excuse for people to blame something that they can claim is beyond their control, in this case their race.

I have three reasons for not believing these BMI-related claims. First, for any one of these racial groups, I have seen multiple examples of members of that group who have adopted a healthy lifestyle and gone from being obese to being a healthy weight. Second, there are a half-dozen people very close to me in my family tree who are or were obese because of a genetic predisposition to obesity. As a consequence, I am strongly genetically predisposed towards obesity. I have fought a constant battle with weight gain every day for over 30 years. Yet I lost weight and have successfully kept it off for more than 30 years, by adopting a healthy lifestyle. Third, if you take a close look at what obese people from these racial groups are actually eating, you soon find that it is food that healthy people do not eat, and in quantities that healthy people do not consume.

You get to choose, and anyone who tells you otherwise is trying to hold you back, hold you down, and take away your opportunities to empower yourself. You need to wrest control away from the naysayers and put it back into your hands, where it belongs. Yes, genetics and metabolism can predispose you towards obesity, but that is no excuse to let them control you, instead of you controlling them!

Let me give a barnyard analogy. Your brain has to take care of your body the same way that a farmer takes care of a barnyard animal. Your brain has to make sure your body gets enough water, gets enough food, has shelter, is transported safely from one place to another, is washed, is clothed, etc.

If you saw a farmer with a goat, and the goat was in the same condition you are in, would you say that that farmer was doing a good job, or would you feel sad for the goat and be reporting the farmer to the authorities for cruelty to animals? With this analogy in mind, take a trip to the shopping mall and look at all the other "farmers" walking about. Are they caring for their bodies in a humane fashion? You have to be committed to caring for your body because it's the only one you'll get!

I told you earlier that I decided that I would rather be hungry all the time than fat all the time. That was a conscious choice. As mentioned earlier, it is such a routine feeling now that my hunger just blends into the background noise. The benefit of my conscious choice is that being hungry all the time means that I can play with my children, go for long walks, jog up the stairs, socialize, mow my lawns, trim my hedges, hold down a stressful job, avoid all sorts of health issues (including sexual health issues), wear normal-sized clothing, fit into an airline seat with space to spare on either side, etc.

Once you choose to give up being fat, you do not have to worry about the lack of strength and lack of mobility that accompany obesity in old age. You don't have to fear the loss of years of life described in Chapter 10. Getting healthy sure beats not being able to put my open hands on my hips, and having stretch marks on my belly.

Speaking of which, after losing weight, I remember the first time I could put my open hands upon my hips/waist. That was the first time in my life I could do it! It felt great. I still get that same great feeling when I put my hands on my hips more than 30 years later.

After losing weight, I remember entering a charity run, and ending in the top 50 runners out of more than a thousand. I even beat a guy I had gone to school with who had been a regional running champion in his day. I saw him again 20 years later and he had gained more weight than I had lost; I did not immediately recognize him, and he did not recognize me at all.

In fact, I often see former athletes who have gained 50 pounds, or 100 pounds. I think three things are going on. First, the former athletes used to consume a high-calorie diet when they were actively engaged in regular sporting activities, and they did not decrease their calorie intake when they stopped being so active. Second, well-known people often have high opinions of themselves and think the usual rules do not apply to them. They do not think about the long-term effects of overeating. It is some sort of sense of entitlement; some sort of blindness to the consequences. Third, well-known people often have a lot of money to spend, even if it is only on credit. So, they tend to eat out frequently at expensive restaurants. The food is not healthy and comes in portions that are too large. Don't act like these people!

Good farmers check their animals regularly.

Getting healthy similarly requires regular monitoring of your body. This is especially true if you gain weight really quickly. My father told me that he wore the same belt all the time, and if it got too tight, that was his signal to eat less and move more. In my case, I use bathroom scales, and, being an MIT geek, I plot the reading on a graph and monitor it. You don't have to go that far, but you do have to monitor yourself.

Overeating takes time, money, and effort. Having to then carry that fat body around takes even more effort. I know how it feels. You could, instead, redirect that effort into something more productive and healthy. Something like walking, or educating yourself about nutrition, or volunteering in your community. Something that constructively redirects and retrains your brain, and gets you moving. Something that engages you with others in your community in a productive fashion. Choose something that counters tendencies toward depression, or guilt, or whatever your particular issue is. Take control now; it's *your* life and *your* choice!

Chapter 8

Body Arithmetic

I published a co-authored research paper in 2015 that was focused on the management of personal credit card debt (Crack and Roberts, 2015). In that research paper, my co-author and I pointed out the similarities between the accumulation of excess financial debt and the accumulation of excess body weight.

For example, both excess financial debt and excess weight are gained slowly over time, and once acquired have to be chipped away at slowly to get back to healthy levels. Also, many people who manage to pay down their debt, subsequently accumulate more debt again, and the same is true of weight loss with yo-yo dieting.

I did not say it in that research paper, but I think that if your life is out of control in one dimension, it is likely out of control in other dimensions too. For example, obese people have lower income, less wealth, and more debt than healthy people (Guthrie and Sokolowsky, 2014).

The symptoms of an unhealthy lifestyle will differ from person to person. Perhaps you spend an unhealthy number of hours in front of a computer screen, or perhaps you buy too many things over the Internet, or perhaps you drink too much, or you never exercise, or you smoke, or your relationships are messed up, or your house is a mess, or your yard is a mess, or your clothes are shabby, or God only knows what else.

Wresting back control of your life is a major goal. It can seem daunting, but remember: it is done in small steps, and it will take time, because whatever your issues are and whatever the symptoms are, it took a long time to get into this situation, and it is going to take a long time, probably years, to get out of it.

Do not expect to solve your problems quickly, because it is not going to happen that way. Your body and mind will fight you every step of the way.

Anything done quickly is unlikely to last, because of homeostasis. Accept now that you are committing to a lifestyle change, not a quick fix. You have to commit to this for the long run.

So, let us talk about gaining weight and losing weight. Let me assume that you are a "slug person." That is, you are someone who does not go out for two-hour walks or out running or have hour-long cardio workouts at the gym, or anything like that. Let me assume that aside from your job (which may be in the home or at an office, etc.), you do not engage in strenuous activity. I call you a slug person because compared with someone following a healthy lifestyle you are a slug.

I have placed my following three-page explanation of body arithmetic between spade symbols to make it stand out. I strongly suspect that most doctors fail to explain this arithmetic to patients either because they condescendingly assume that their patients are not intelligent enough to understand it, or because they do not understand it themselves (doctors are notoriously bad at even basic math). Doctors would rather give up on you and recommend a pill or surgery than take the time to explain this to you! So, please read it slowly and carefully, and reread it if it is not clear.

♠ Suppose you are at a healthy weight and you want to gain 45 pounds and keep it on forever. What should you do? Yes, I said *gain*. If we talk about that first, it will help you to understand how your body works.

A simple way to gain 45 pounds is to eat one extra average-sized banana a day over and above your body's calorie needs, and to do that for only five years in a row. You will gain about four-tenths of an ounce in weight a day, and over five years, that adds up to just over 45 pounds extra weight in total. Then to keep that extra 45 pounds and gain no more, all you have to do is stop eating that extra banana each day. (Note that I am not suggesting that bananas are unhealthy; they are just a common food group that most folks can relate to.)

This example is interesting for two reasons. First, it takes very little extra food each day to gain 45 pounds in only five years. Anything with the equivalent calories to an average banana will do the job. That's really important because maybe you buy one of those calorie-laden coffees at lunch, or maybe you have an extra half a muffin, or equivalent, at dessert. It might not seem like much, but it adds up to a significant amount in a relatively short time span. Homeostasis will not protect you, because you are fooling your body into accepting this weight gain slowly over time.

Second, if after having gained the 45 pounds, you then remove the extra daily banana over and above your body's calorie needs, then this just brings your consumption back to your body's daily calorie needs. If from then on you consume only what your body needs, you will neither gain weight nor lose it. You will hold onto those extra 45 pounds until you die. So, in this case, cutting out that extra food does not lead to a weight loss. This is really important: If you are currently consuming above your body's calorie needs, then reducing your calorie intake might not lead to any weight loss.

For example, if you are consuming one banana per day over your body's calorie needs, and you cut out only the equivalent of half a banana a day, say, then even though you have reduced your calorie intake, you will still be gaining weight—because you are still consuming a half banana more than your body's daily energy requirements.

For some folks (for example, the birthday boy in Davis I mentioned previously), the energy gap is enormous, and even if they cut out a significant amount of food they may still gain weight. Some of these folks tried that already in an attempt to lose weight, and gave up when they failed, not realizing that they were still consuming more calories than their body needed, even after the reduction in their intake. It is simple body arithmetic.

Let me assume again that you are a slug person. I told you already that if you eat one extra banana a day over and above your body's daily energy needs, then this energy gap means that you will gain 45 pounds of excess weight in five years. I also told you that if you then eliminate the extra banana, and bring your calorie intake down to your body's actual needs, you will hold onto that extra 45 pounds until you drop dead.

If, however, after gaining the 45 pounds, you eliminate that one extra banana a day, and also eliminate an additional second banana's worth of other food intake, then you will create a negative energy gap. That is, you will be one banana short of your body's daily energy requirements. This energy gap will require that your body burn the extra fat store that you are carrying. You will lose about four-tenths of an ounce per day, and after five years, you will have lost the entire 45 pounds. At that stage, you can increase your consumption back to your body's needs, adding back roughly one banana per day, and then maintain the weight loss. ♠

I cannot overemphasize the importance of the above explanation. If you did not understand it, then stop reading now. Go back three pages and reread the material between the spade symbols as many times as it takes until you fully understand it.

If you are young and fat, do not assume that you need to do nothing about it. **If you are already fat, then you have clearly been consuming more than your body's daily calorie needs. Continuing to do so will just steadily pack on extra pounds.** Now is the time to address this problem, take control, and reverse the trend. To do so, however, you need to know your body's energy needs.

Unfortunately, your body's energy needs are difficult to measure. I like to think of it as a relatively constant number (see the "delicate equilibrium" argument below), but in fact it is a very slowly changing number. As we age, for example, our body's energy needs tend to fall. If we exercise more, or go through a very stressful life-changing event, our body's energy needs increase, etc. The simplest way to think about it is in relative terms. If you eat more than your body needs right now, then you will surely gain weight, and if you eat less than your body needs right now, then you will surely lose weight. There is no other possibility.

Let us go back to the 45-pound-overweight example. Suppose that you can cut out that extra banana per day, but that for some other reasons you simply cannot cut out a second banana's worth of food intake per day. If you stop right there, you will not lose a pound. Your body will hold on to every ounce of it. Well, then the obvious thing to do is substitute that additional reduction in calorie intake with an extra banana's worth of exercise per day. An extra banana's worth of exercise per day will have exactly the same effect as cutting out a banana's worth of food.

How much exercise do you have to do per day to equate to a banana's worth of food intake? One banana's worth of calories equates almost exactly to a brisk one-mile walk (or a slightly less-than-one-mile jog). A healthy person can walk one mile in 20 minutes, but it might take you longer.

Now, my example above is for someone 45 pounds overweight who is currently eating only one banana a day over his or her body's daily energy needs. If you are 90 pounds overweight and eating only one banana a day over your body's daily energy needs, then the story is similar. Cut out one banana's worth of food per day, and you will hold onto every ounce. Cut out two bananas' worth of food per day, however, and you will lose four-tenths of an ounce per day, and in 10 years' time you will have lost the full 90 pounds. Can you check my arithmetic?

How much over your body's daily energy needs are you consuming? I fear, unfortunately, that for many people this energy gap is way more than a single banana. The only way for you to find this out for sure is to experiment with a slow, day-by-day reduction in your food intake, and an accompanying increase in your exercise, until your frequent weigh-ins begin to show a sure sign of weight loss. Once you start losing weight, then you need to stick to that regime (or a more serious regime) until you reach a healthy weight (or a realistic goal weight).

Do you think 10 years sounds like a long time? Do you think that you do not have the patience to stick with it? Well, let me tell you something. Stop it right now! You are being dishonest with yourself. If you think that healthy weight loss and attaining a healthy weight is something you can do in less than a year, then either you are living in la-la land, or you are being dishonest with yourself.

If you honestly want to achieve a healthy weight

and maintain that healthy weight, then you need to make a commitment to doing so, and you need to accept the truth: you are fat and unhealthy, and you did not get this way overnight. So, getting healthy is going to take almost as long as getting unhealthy took, and it is going to be hard work all the way. You overate almost every day to get to where you are; now you need to under-eat every day to get back again. If you try to do this quickly, then homeostasis will kick you back to where you are now, by definition. You have to put in the hard work to reach the goal. It is time for honesty and a commitment. If you think you have it tough, then, as FDR said, go tell that to the Marines!

Let me tell you, however, that there is some light at the end of the tunnel. If you under-eat for the next however many years it takes to reach your healthy weight, then when you reach that target you will be able to increase your calorie intake. In fact, you are going to have to, or else you will waste away to nothing. By then you should have a good idea of your body's energy needs, and with frequent weigh-ins, you should be able to quickly respond if you find yourself gaining weight again. You cannot, however, return to the calorie intake you have now, or you will just get fat and unhealthy again.

As you get healthier, you will almost certainly gain muscle mass. Muscles weigh more than fat and burn more calories than fat. So, you may gain weight (in the form of muscle mass) in order to help lose weight (in the form of fat). Indeed, adding some load-bearing exercises (carrying or lifting weights) to your routine can accelerate your muscle gain. Yes, even young women should aim to gain some muscle mass. Don't worry, you are not going to look like some freaky body builder.

Creatine monohydrate is a popular supplement that can help you gain muscle mass. If you begin taking creatine, you may gain an immediate 3–6 pounds. That gain in muscle weight will help you work off the fat and get healthy. Again, this is a reminder that weight loss is not the goal. Some people, however, cannot take creatine because it makes them jumpy.

There is a delicate equilibrium at work, presided over by your brain and by homeostasis. When you carry your overweight body around, you burn more calories than a person carrying a healthy-weight body around—because you are carrying an extra load they are not carrying. As you lose fat, however, other things being equal, your body does not need to burn as many calories as it did previously to carry your extra load around, and your body's energy needs drop. Other things are not equal, however, because as you exercise and gain muscle mass, you need to support that exercise and feed those muscles, which increases your body's calorie needs. So, weighing all these factors up, it may be that as you become healthier, your body's daily energy needs do not change much at all.

(Do you think that is all too much information? Well, this is the reality of weight loss logic that doctors either do not understand themselves or judge you not intelligent enough to understand. You deserve better! You deserve to know all the facts so that you can make informed choices.)

Although I said that your body's daily energy needs may be relatively constant, there are exceptions, of course. When I was in the final year of my PhD studies at MIT, I went through a period of several months where I was working 135 hours per week, rather than my normal 80–100 hours per week (I kept a timesheet religiously). I was doing at least one all-nighter per week, and often a double all-nighter instead or as well (a double all-nighter is when you go to work at 7 A.M. Monday and work through until 11 P.M. Wednesday, say). With the long hours of work and little sleep, I'd wake up suddenly on the subway at midnight, or in the bathtub (because the water got cold), or sitting at my computer with the keyboard overload alarm going off (because I went to sleep with my hands on the keyboard). With all the associated stress and brain work, I was eating five meals a day but still losing weight.

(As an aside, you could argue that regularly working over 100 hours per week was not a healthy activity and that it is hypocritical behavior from the author of a book about getting healthy, and you would be right. At MIT, however, it seemed perfectly normal to play Frisbee with classmates at 3 A.M. after working a 45-hour day, go home and get two hours sleep, then work an 18-hour day, have a 10-mile run and a hot shower, then get another few hours' sleep, and then go and do another all-nighter, etc. This was an exceptional time in my life, and I am trying to make the point that during exceptional times your calorie intake may increase dramatically.)

Similarly, pregnant women need extra calories, and people recovering from injuries need extra calories to heal. In general, stressful or busy periods temporarily increase your body's calorie needs. You need to monitor yourself to make sure you neither overeat nor get depleted.

The bottom line is that you need to understand basic body arithmetic and you need to make a commitment to monitoring your body's reaction to calorie intake and exercise, adjusting these as necessary to stay on the path to getting healthy.

Chapter 9

Exercise

Look back 100 years, and you will likely find that many of your ancestors worked on a farm, or as a housewife, or in a mill, or in a dockyard, or down a mine, or in the military, or laboring, or something similar. They did not have cars. They did not have supermarkets. There was no Internet shopping. Exercise was what they did while they were working. They could not do their jobs if they were unhealthy. They went home tired from physical exertion. They were fit and strong and they slept well.

Nowadays, many people are much more sedentary than they were 100 years ago. Many of us work long hours at a desk, or at some manual labor job that is not very taxing. We drive to the supermarket and fill our shopping cart.

Making time for exercise is difficult, and doing so means that something else has to give. Maybe you are going to get behind on the laundry, or your house won't be spotless, or you cannot go out and socialize as often as you'd like. Fitting in exercise and giving up something else in exchange may add stress to your life, even though exercise is meant to be a de-stressor!

The 1996 U.S. Surgeon General's report on physical activity says that significant health benefits can be obtained by including a moderate amount of physical activity on most, if not all, days of the week (U.S. Department of Health and Human Services, 1996, p. 4). The report suggests 30 minutes of brisk walking or 15 minutes of running per day, or something similar. It goes on to say, however, that despite "common knowledge that exercise is healthful, more than 60 percent of American adults are not regularly active, and 25 percent of the adult population are not active at all (U.S. Department of Health and Human Services, 1996, p. 5)."

Similarly, the U.K. National Health Service Physical Activity Guidelines recommend that adults do at least 150 minutes of moderate-intensity aerobic activity every week (that is, about 20 minutes per day) along with muscle-strengthening exercises twice a week, or, alternatively, 75 minutes of vigorous intensity activity per week (that is, about 10 minutes per day), or something similar (NHS, 2011). A 2013 study in the U.K., with a sample of over 1 million persons, found, however, that only one in five people in England met the guidelines for moderate physical activity (Farrell et al., 2013, Table 1).

When I was a PhD student, I knew a fellow I will call "Jack," who was the nicest guy in the world. Jack went out of his way to help me with my work and I thanked him for it. Jack was obese, and fully aware of it. He knew that I exercised a lot and he declared to me once that he hated exercise with a passion, and he meant it. He was very intelligent, and I think that he was honest with himself. He knew he was obese, and he chose not to do anything about it. I do wonder, however, whether he realized how short his life was going to be as a consequence. I was very sad to see Jack's death reported when he was barely 50. (See also the statistics on life expectancy in Chapter 10.)

To avoid such a dreadful outcome, you need to

combine calorie reduction with healthy food choices and additional exercise. If weight loss were the only goal, then calorie reduction or additional exercise alone would suffice, if done in sufficient quantity, but weight loss is not the goal. The goal is getting healthy and thereby achieving a healthy weight. So, you need to reduce calories, make healthy food choices, and exercise more.

Should you jump in the deep end and go from being overweight and never exercising properly to trying to run five miles every day? No, of course not. That's ridiculous! Your body will give up within 48 hours. You will have blisters on your feet and pain in your joints, and your brain will tell you in no uncertain terms to stop what you are doing.

Like everything else, your exercise routine has to be introduced gently to fool your brain and your body into accepting it as the new normal. Otherwise, homeostasis will kick in to defeat you.

I recommend that you start with walking. If you must include running, then for goodness' sake start slowly! You can walk 100 yards, then jog 50 yards slowly, then walk another 100 yards, and jog 50 yards slowly, and so on. Alternatively, you can walk four lampposts, then jog to the next one, then walk another four, and so on. Be sure to pace yourself!

If you start with walking only, then how far should you walk? Start with around the block. If that is fine, then try two times around the block tomorrow. If that is fine, then try three times around the block the day after. Increase it every day until you know your limits.

Don't worry about how you look—you look better exercising than you do sitting on the sofa! People who understand your battle will respect your efforts; people who do not respect your efforts are naysayers, and you do not care what they think.

In my office building, I see plenty of folks who choose to walk up the stairs, or they take the elevator a floor or two, and then walk the rest of the way, or they walk part way and take the elevator the rest of the way. If that suits you, then do so whenever possible.

Note that if you are fat, then you are heavy. If you have not exercised much lately, then your feet are likely too soft to walk much without protection. So, you need a pair of comfortable athletic shoes.

You also need to get some athletic medical tape from the drug store ($5 worth of tape will last six months probably). The tape is usually about one to one-and-one-half inches wide, sticky, light brown, and made with a cloth-like texture. The kind that you can tear with your hands is better than the kind that you have to cut with scissors.

Put tape on the tops of your toes, the sides of your feet, sensitive parts of your soles, and your heels—like a boxer taping his hands before a fight. Do not cut off any circulation in the process. The tape may stay in place for a week before it needs replacing; don't tear it off early because it will take skin with it. It can get wet in the shower and still stick, so leave it in place until it is falling off. It's not meant to be pretty; it's meant to reduce the likelihood of blisters, injury, and pain. It's meant to keep you moving.

You might not realize it, but most of the folks you see out running in the street have their feet taped up. Otherwise, they would be getting home with blisters and a sock full of blood after each run. You do not want sore or blistered feet to be yet another excuse for not getting healthy; we have had enough of excuses. So, protect yourself by anticipating this problem with small patches of tape on the areas of your feet most likely to chafe. If you notice anywhere else chafing or getting damaged, then put protection there too; white petroleum jelly may be useful for noses, ears, and toes in the winter.

Get a light waterproof outer shell ($30 at your

local outdoors shop). You are going to need it on rainy days, and it helps if it is light for rainy summer days. Bad weather is no excuse!

I have been out walking or running in deep snow, heavy hail, torrential rain, high winds, $-20\,°F$ with icicles forming on my eyebrows, $+95\,°F$ where I am sweating bullets, etc. The only weather conditions in which I would not go out for a walk or run is during the height of a thunderstorm when there are lightning bolts visibly cracking the air, if it is below about $-20\,°F$, or if there is violent surface flooding.

Once you know how far you can walk, use that distance to explore your city. When I moved to the Boston area, I was running 10 miles three times a week. I used that to explore my city. I went all over the place at all hours of the day and night, including unsafe places you should not go—but at least I was running, so when people chased me, they could not catch me!

When I moved to London, I would use the Tube and my feet to get to work. I lived in the West End, but worked in the City (that is, in East London). So, I got to explore almost everything in-between on foot. If I walked halfway to work, I would take the Tube the rest of the way. If I took the Tube half way, I would walk the remainder. With London's old and narrow network of streets, I could walk a different way every day.

I cannot emphasize how much more you see on foot that you ever do in a car or a bus. I discovered unusual places that nobody else seemed to know about. My London firm was headquartered in San Francisco. So, I got to know those streets too. Jogging in Paris on holidays in France means that I also got to know downtown Paris quite well.

As a tourist in these cities nowadays, the unusual places I discovered previously are now my favorite places to visit. I exploit my very detailed knowledge of the streets of Boston, London, San Francisco, and Paris whenever I travel. When mistaken for a resident of these cities, I can almost always give directions to lost tourists or business people—all because of a committed choice made just over 30 years ago.

Of course, there are downsides to running. One downside is that whatever you ate for breakfast and lunch gets shaken 10,000 times when you go for an afternoon run, like putting the food in a blender. This doesn't happen when you walk. So, you need to time your runs with that in mind. Choose your food carefully (for example, I discovered that I cannot eat apples, apricots, or oranges during the 18 hours before a long run).

Another downside of running is that it is much easier to get injured running that walking. I have had some serious running injuries where I impacted something, or something impacted me. These would never have happened had I been walking.

Yet another downside of running is that people shout out abuse at me or throw things at me when I am running pretty much every week. They shout insults, sexual comments, or just plain crazy stuff. They throw beer bottles, beer cans, eggs, snow balls or ice balls (in the winter), cups of water, garbage, etc. On multiple occasions, I have had people spit at me from windows and balconies while shouting abuse. Some shouted comments are, however, funny or good natured ("Run, Forrest, Run" or "give me a high five!"), but some are downright nasty. I suspect that young women who go jogging receive just as much abuse as I do, but my guess is that a larger proportion of it is likely to be of a sexual nature.

The majority of these abusive events happened while running in N.Z. When running in the U.K. and France, I never took any abuse at all; in Paris almost nobody runs, and I think folks assumed I must be a firefighter or in the military. When running in the U.S., the abuse I have attracted has typically been of a uniformly nasty sort, including racial insults, verbal threats of physical violence, and people trying to physically attack me.

On the plus side, when you go running, you join a community of runners. In N.Z., any runner can say hello to any other runner while out running, regardless of gender, age, racial group, etc. That's not necessarily true on the East Coast of the U.S., but it holds in many places I have been.

I guess the bottom line is that after running well in excess of 30,000 miles (more than 50,000 kilometers), bad things are bound to have happened sometimes. The frequency no longer surprises me. My advice is to stick to well-lit and well-populated areas during daylight hours, have a plan in mind for when people insult you or attempt to assault you, and always keep some energy in reserve so you can sprint out of danger when you need to (once you are fit, your attackers will likely be less fit than you!).

Although I have had my share of bad experiences when running, running still suits me, even in my 50s, but it is certainly not for everyone. Quite frankly, swift walking would bring me many of the same benefits and save many of the costs that running brings. So, I recommend walking to start with, and you may never get to running, depending upon your brain and body.

Is exercise fun and exciting? No, after 30 years of regular exercise, I have no conclusion other than that exercise is boring and time consuming. Yes, maybe you can watch a movie while working out at the gym, or talk to a friend while speed walking, or maybe you can walk somewhere interesting when vacationing in Paris. Most of the time, however, you are on your own (because you simply cannot rely upon anyone but yourself to be there), and you are exercising for such long time periods and so frequently that it is just plain boring. Don't expect it to be exciting or interesting.

Let me discuss a related point. My friends and family members often remark upon the fact that I both eat far less than they do, and exercise far more than they do, in order to have roughly the same silhouette that they already have. I suspect that the fact that I am strongly genetically predisposed towards obesity means that my body uses its calories more efficiently than the average person's body does. Perhaps you and I are descended from hunters who used to run long distances to catch prey (or something like that), and our metabolisms are slow and particularly efficient, burning calories at a slower rate than other folks doing the same work. So, when we eat like normal folk and exercise only a little, we quickly get fat. I fear that the simple fact that you are fat means that you, like me, may require much more exercise than the average person in order to be healthy. Unfortunately, this predisposition will make exercise all the more time consuming for you.

One positive aspect of the time-consuming nature of exercise is that it gives you ample time to think about things. When I am running, I always have a pen and paper in my pocket. I use them to jot down notes about anything that occurs to me while running (ideas for a book, solutions to work-related problems, the realization that I did not pay my taxes yet, etc.).

One way to look at this boring, time-consuming side of exercise is that you can spend time doing your exercise now, or you can spend time in doctors' offices later. Indeed, I have seen many unhealthy people who seem to have made a career out of doctors' visits, hospital visits, and surgeries.

My jaded view is that it takes time to eat yourself into an unhealthy situation. This then leads to still more time spent with health professionals, many of whom can do very little to address any of your subsequent issues. So much wasted time!

The other side of the coin is, as mentioned above, that if you instead spend time exercising now, then that is an investment you make that removes the need to spend time with health professionals later. You won't need to see them as often as other less healthy people do. At the same time, you are also buying extra time in retirement (to travel, visit grandchildren, draw on your pension, etc.). The unhealthy people will not get this extra time because they will be dead or disabled.

I have seen some exercise machines advertised with the tagline that they require only a four-minute workout per day. I have seen friends who insist that their very short power workout at the gym takes care of all their exercise needs. These "workouts" are fads. They are not healthy. Your ancestors spent long periods of time performing physical labor. You cannot replace three hours chasing an antelope or eight hours down a coal mine with four minutes on some shiny machine. Exercise is time consuming and boring. It's like going to work at a job you hate but which pays you money you desperately need, or like taking a dose of essential medicine every day. You simply don't have a choice if you want to live.

It may seem a long way off, but once your weight reaches a relatively healthy level, you need to be careful not to exercise too much. Once your fat stores are reduced, you need to be sure that you eat enough to avoid physical collapse. It can be difficult to get the balance just right.

I think that the healthy choice is to be a little overweight. That way, you have some fat reserves in place in case you get sick, injured, or exercise too much. If you are underweight, then you risk damaging yourself when you need to call upon the reserves you do not have.

For example, I have often seen very thin young women out jogging who clearly need to increase their calorie intakes. Sure enough, they are not fat, but neither are they healthy. They look as if they have been on a starvation diet in some prison camp. No way could they sprint if they needed too. No way could they fight off an attacker. They need to eat more, exercise less, and gain weight to get to a healthy weight. Again, this is a reminder that weight loss is not the goal.

The bottom line is that you should understand and monitor the effect of exercise on your body from now until the day you attain a healthy weight, and for the rest of your life afterwards.

Chapter 10

Time Machine

Eating too much, eating unhealthy foods, and not exercising are, when taken together, a form of short-sighted risk taking. They betray a lack of foresight or a lack of imagination on your part. It would be helpful to be able to step into a time machine and to be able to see the future consequences of your actions.

So, I want to give you some insight into the future you want to avoid by looking at two different time machines. Each "time machine" is, in fact, a scientific study that enables me to look into your future and see what your life will be like if you do not get healthy. The first study (actually a series of studies) deals with overlapping health-related and retirement-related issues, and the second study deals with life expectancy and lost quality of life issues.

I am going to jump straight to the conclusions, and then you can either read the rest of this chapter for the details that back up my forecasts, or you can skip over them and go straight to the last two paragraphs of this chapter.

Based on the following two time machines, if you have chosen to be obese, then I forecast that you will fall into the half the population that has to **retire earlier than planned because of health-related issues**, and I predict that you will **not be able to work in retirement**. When your early retirement comes, you will **not have saved enough money to be comfortable in retirement**. On top of this, if you are 20–39 years old, say, then you can expect that your **decision to be obese will rob you of between four and seven years of life** (compared with a healthy-weight person), and that during your remaining years of life **you will lose an additional 10 to 17 years of healthy life** (compared with a healthy-weight person). This is your future if you do nothing about your health issues. Fortunately, you get to choose.

Time Machine #1: Retirement

Each year, the Employee Benefit Research Institute (EBRI) conducts a Retirement Confidence Survey (RCS) in the U.S. My guess is that you have never heard of it, even though the EBRI has been doing it for 25 years, and it is the longest-running annual retirement survey of its kind in the U.S.

Usually folks switch off when they hear the words "retirement" or "survey," but let me tell you why the RCS is vitally important to you.

The EBRI goes out and asks pre-retirees about what they *think* is going to happen in their future lives, and then they ask retirees about what *actually* happened. The EBRI talks to people just like you. So, looking at the survey results gives you the opportunity to look at potential outcomes for yourself in a kind of time machine. The results are consistently and predictably shocking.

Let me take the average of several recent EBRI surveys (Helman et al., 2015; Helman et al., 2014, 2013) and smudge the results slightly to make them easier to understand.

The EBRI finds that roughly three out of every four pre-retirees (people in their 50s) plan to work in retirement. Almost everyone who says they are planning to work in retirement gives a financial reason for doing so, but they invariably give non-financial reasons too (like staying engaged with people, having something to do, etc.).

For the most part, however, these pre-retirees (folks just like you perhaps?) are fooling themselves. What actually happens is that roughly only one in four retirees actually ends up working in retirement. The big difference between expectations of pre-retirees and outcomes of actual retirees is that two out of every four people have to retire earlier than they planned and are unable to work in retirement.

There are a number of reasons given in the surveys for leaving the workforce earlier than planned, but the most common reason by far is health and disability (around 60 percent of people leaving the workforce early give this reason). Another very common reason for a worker leaving the workforce early is that the health of their spouse failed, and they have to look after their spouse (around 20 percent of people leaving the workforce early give this reason).

Unfortunately, the people who retired sooner than planned invariably state that they are less confident about having saved enough money for retirement. Why is this? Well, suppose that you are planning to work in retirement, and that you have a financial reason for doing so, but then your health or the health of your spouse fails. This means that not only do you not get to work in retirement as previously planned, but on top of that you have to stop work before a traditional retirement date.

So, you get hit with the double whammy of missing out on both the money you were going to make working up until your planned retirement date and the extra money you were planning on making in retirement. No wonder these folks leaving the workforce early are less confident than others about their retirement savings! Quite frankly, none of these results should be surprising.

Time Machine #2: Years of Life

The second time machine I want to look at allows you to forecast the impact of being fat on life expectancy (that is, lost years of life) and on quality of life (that is, lost healthy years of life, where a healthy year of life is defined as a remaining year of life that is free from cardiovascular disease and diabetes).

I could have filled 100 pages with the results of

100 different research papers supporting the argument that being fat is bad for you. For example, the list of cancers related to being fat is long and convincing in both males and females (Parkin, D.M., and L. Boyd, 2011). I think, however, that many people ignore cancer risk. So, by focusing instead on lost years of life and lost years of healthy life, I may have a greater impact on your actions.[1] So, I have chosen one recent paper that has results which are particularly clear and compelling in this respect.

Grover et al. (2015) used a sample of roughly 4,000 people. Their sample was roughly half male and half female, and their results were about the same for both genders. Their results were different, however, depending upon your age and whether you are overweight, obese, or very obese.

---

[1] If you are, however, interested in cancer risks more generally, I strongly recommend the easy-to-understand summary table appearing in WCRF/AICR (2007, p. 370). It shows convincing and probable factors that increase or decrease many different cancer risks and obesity risks. **Physical activity, breastfeeding, and eating fruit and non-starchy vegetables top the list for decreasing your risks. Body fatness, drinking alcohol, and abdominal fatness top the list for increasing your risks.** Note that smoking is conspicuously absent from the summary table as a cancer risk, because there is no doubt whatsoever that it is the chief cause of lung cancer (WCRF/AICR, 2007, p. xxiii).

As you would expect, if you are fat, then you are straining and abusing your body's health. The younger you acquire that fat, or the more fat that you acquire, then the more strain/abuse your body is subject to, and the worse the impact on your life expectancy and on the risk of an early onset of cardiovascular disease and diabetes. (As an aside, the authors also find that the impact of being fat is worse in non-smokers than smokers. The simple explanation is that smokers have proportionately less life ahead of them than non-smokers, and choosing to be fat during that shorter life therefore has a proportionally lesser impact on lost years.)

The study contains many detailed results (Grover et al., 2015, Figure 2). Let me, however, give ranges of likely forecast outcomes, and let me smudge the results slightly to make them easier to understand.

- If you are **young** (that is, 20–39 years old), Grover et al. (2015) find that being **overweight** robs you of about 1–4 years of life, and an additional 5–8 years of healthy life; being **obese** robs you of about 4–7 years of life, and an additional 10–17 years of healthy life; and being **very obese** robs you of about 5–10 years of life, and an additional 17–22 years of healthy life.

- If you are **middle-aged** (that is, 40–59 years old), being **overweight** robs you of about 1–2 years of life, and an additional 1–5 years of healthy life; being **obese** robs you of about 1–4 years of life, and an additional 5–12 years of healthy life; and being **very obese** robs you of about 2–6 years of life, and an additional 10–18 years of healthy life.

- If you are **older** (that is, 60–79 years old), being **overweight** robs you of about 1–2 years of life, and an additional 0–4 years of healthy life; being **obese** robs you of about 0–2 years of life, and an additional 2–7 years of healthy life; and being **very obese** robs you of about 0–2 years of life, and an additional 3–9 years of healthy life.

Just as with my first time machine, there is a double whammy here. Not only does being fat mean that you can expect to live fewer years, it also means that that during your remaining years, you can expect to experience more unhealthy years than a healthy-weight person. Again, quite frankly, none of these results should be surprising.

Based on the above two time machines and on discussions in the previous chapters, if you have chosen to be obese, then it will not surprise me at all to find that your spouse (if you have one) is also obese. As mentioned already, I forecast that you will fall into the half the population that has to retire early because of health issues, and I predict that you will not be able to work in retirement. I assume that when your early retirement comes, you will not have saved enough money to be comfortable in retirement. On top of this, if you are 20–39 years old, say, you can expect that your decision to be obese will rob you of between four and seven years of life (compared with a healthy-weight person), and that during your remaining years of life you will lose an additional 10 to 17 years of healthy life (compared with a healthy-weight person). This is your future if you do nothing about your health issues.

These are terrible and sobering outcomes. They carry with them many other impacts, like not having enough money to travel once retired, losing your mobility at an early age, torturing your body with a drug cocktail prescribed by doctors who have essentially given up on you, not being alive to see your grandchildren graduate from college, etc. These terrible outcomes are all avoidable. You get to choose!

In the last chapter I summarize the main points of the book.

Conclusion

Let me now bring together the main points from the previous chapters. Look back through the book, or use the index to find more detail on any of these main points.

- This book is about empowerment, being committed, and making powerful choices. You can choose to not be fat any more, educate yourself, and then execute your choice. It is going to be hard work but you are worth it.

- Weight loss is not the goal, and aiming for weight loss typically fails. The goal is getting healthy, and thereby attaining a healthy weight.

- If you are fat, then embrace that fact instead of trying to hide it. It is liberating to say "I am fat, and I'm sick and tired of it" out loud.

- Making powerful choices is itself empowering, and doors start opening for you once you do so.

- Your body is a complicated biological machine, but it is a machine nevertheless. A negative energy gap means that you must lose weight. A positive energy gap means that you must gain weight. It is simple body arithmetic.

- You need to impose limits on what you eat and when you eat. You need to monitor your weight regularly.

- You need to exercise more, but homeostasis will stop your mind and body from accepting dramatic changes in exercise routines. So, introduce exercise slowly to your daily routine.

- Exercise is often boring and time consuming. Exercise is like working at a job you hate but which you need to survive.

- There are many techniques for getting healthy that fool your body into accepting fewer calories, and that fly under the radar of homeostasis.

- You are reading this book because you have underlying issues. Life may have dealt you a lousy hand, but you need to be honest about your issues, and commit to addressing them.

- Confront your issues head on, on your terms. Exercise, and getting healthy, helps to address many issues.

- If you act like a victim, you will be a victim. If you adopt a winning mindset and fight obesity, then you can win the battle. Refuse to lose!

- If you are fat, then you have been consuming more than your body's daily calorie needs. Continuing to do so will just steadily pack on extra pounds.

- I chose to be hungry all the time instead of being fat all the time. Being hungry all the time is an unpleasant feeling, but it is a better feeling than the feeling of being fat all the time. After a while, feeling hungry just becomes routine and that feeling fades into the background noise.

- You get to choose a healthy life, and anyone who tells you otherwise is trying to hold you back, hold you down, and take away your opportunities to empower yourself. You must fight them.

- Stop looking for crutches. Look inwards. You, and only you, control what you eat and how and when you exercise. Be there for yourself 24-7.

- Recognize fad diets as unhealthy. For example, no healthy diet demonizes entire food groups. If you need structure, find it in reduced calorie intake, regular meal times, and a regular exercise routine, not in the crazy strictures of some fad diet.

- Don't blame your metabolism. Sure enough, your metabolism may be slow, but that's no excuse! That's just shifting the blame. It is *your* brain lifting *your* arm to put *your* choice of food (quantity and quality) into *your* mouth. It is *your* brain not taking *your* body out for exercise. There is nothing else and nobody else to blame, but you.

- Restaurant food is treat food. Reduce restaurant visits to no more than once or twice per month.

- Don't smoke, use excessive salt, or drink sweetened sodas. These are not part of a healthy life.

- Alcohol is very caloric. Reduce alcohol consumption.

- Breastfeeding is part of a healthy choice for mother and child. Healthy choices also have community benefits that reflect your patriotism.

- AAP Policy Statement: Exclusive breastfeeding for roughly six months is sufficient for optimal growth and development of your child, and continued breastfeeding should take place until at least 12 months of age, and after that for as long as mutually desired by mother and child (Gartner et al., 2005; Eidelman and Schanler, 2012).

- Beware of your membership in affinity groups that adopt unhealthy lifestyles (ethnic groups, religious groups, work groups, etc.). Be a leader in your group, promoting healthy changes, not a follower.

- If you are obese and do nothing about it, it is easy to predict that your life will have terrible and sobering outcomes. You will retire sooner than planned and have less money saved for retirement than planned. You will lose years of life and also years of healthy life. These dire outcomes are avoidable.

Now is the time to become empowered. Now is the time to make your powerful choice. Invest the time now so that you can replace an unhealthy future with an increasingly healthy future. Insure yourself against common bad outcomes by committing to getting healthy and attaining a healthy weight. Make *your* powerful choice now. It is you, and only you, who can make this choice, and I wish you every success. I know you can do it.

Finally, let me repeat my plea from the beginning of the book. If after reading this book and making the sorts of personal choices I describe, you find that your health and quality of life improves, then please go to `Amazon.com` and leave a positive review for this book so that other people may similarly benefit from it. Just type the ISBN number from the back cover into Amazon's Web site and then click on the box labeled "Write a customer review." Thank you.

References

Agarwal, Sanjiv, Carroll Reider, James R. Brooks, and Victor L. Fulgoni, 2015, "Comparison of Prevalence of Inadequate Nutrient Intake Based on Body Weight Status of Adults in the United States: An Analysis of NHANES 20012008," *Journal of the American College of Nutrition*, Vol. 34 No. 2, (April), pp. 126–134.

Berg, Christina, and Heléne Bertéus Forslund, 2015, "The Influence of Portion Size and Timing of Meals on Weight Balance and Obesity," *Current Obesity Reports*, Vol. 4 No. 1, (January), pp. 11–18.

Biesiekierski, Jessica R., Simone L. Peters, Evan D. Newnham, Ourania Rosella, Jane G. Muir, and Peter R. Gibson, 2013, "No Effects of Gluten in Patients with Self-Reported Non-Celiac Gluten Sensitivity after Dietary Reduction of Fermentable, Poorly Absorbed, Short-Chain Carbohydrates," *Gastroenterology*, Vol. 145 No. 2, (August), pp. 320–328.

BLS, 2014, "Women in the Labor Force: A Databook," U.S. Bureau of Labor Statistics, Report 1049, (May), 106 pp.

Bolton, Paul, 2012, "Education: Historical statistics," House of Commons Library, Social & General Statistics, Standard Note: SN/SG/4252, (27 November), 20 pp.

Crack, Timothy Falcon, and Helen M. Roberts, 2015, "Credit Cards, Excess Debt, and the Time Value of Money: The Parable of the Debt Banana," *The Journal of Financial Education*, Vol. 41 No. 1, (Spring), pp. 117–137.

Eidelman, Arthur I., and Richard J. Schanler; (American Academy of Pediatrics Section on Breastfeeding), 2012, "Policy Statement: Breastfeeding and the Use of Human Milk," *Pediatrics*, Vol. 129 No. 3, (March), pp. e827–e841.

Esterl, Mike, 2015, "Soft Drinks Hit 10th Year of Decline: Diet Soda Volumes Fall Sharply, Bottled Water Makes Gains," *The Wall Street Journal Online*, March 26, 2015, Available at: http://www.wsj.com/articles/pepsi-cola-replaces-diet-coke-as-no-2-soda-1427388559 (dated March 26, 2015; downloaded July 2015).

Farrell, Lisa, Bruce Hollingsworth, Carol Propper, and Michael A. Shields, 2013, The Socioeconomic Gradient in Physical Inactivity in England, Working Paper

No. 13/311, Centre for Market and Public Organisation, University of Bristol, (July), 33 pp.

Fasano, Alessio Anna Sapone, Victor Zevallos, and Detlef Schuppan, 2015, "Nonceliac Gluten Sensitivity," *Gastroenterology*, Vol. 148 No. 6, (May), pp. 1195–1204.

Foterek, Kristina, Annett Hilbig, and Ute Alexy, 2014, "Breast-Feeding and Weaning Practices in the DONALD Study: Age and Time Trends," *Journal of Pediatric Gastroenterology and Nutrition*, Vol. 58 No. 3, (March), pp. 361–367.

Garfield, Alastair S., Chia Li, Joseph C. Madara, Bhavik P. Shah, Emily Webber, Jennifer S. Steger, John N. Campbell, Oksana Gavrilova, Charlotte E. Lee, David P. Olson, Joel K. Elmquist, Bakhos A. Tannous, Michael J. Krashes, and Bradford B. Lowell, 2015, "A Neural Basis for Melanocortin-4 ReceptorRegulated Appetite," *Nature Neuroscience*, Vol. 18 No. 6, (27 April), pp. 863–871.

Gartner, Lawrence M., Jane Morton, Ruth A. Lawrence, Audrey J. Naylor, Donna O'Hare, Richard J. Schanler, and Arthur I. Eidelman; (American Academy of Pediatrics Section on Breastfeeding), 2005, "Policy Statement: Breastfeeding and the Use of Human Milk," *Pediatrics*, Vol. 115 No. 2, (February), pp. 496–506.

Green, Peter H.R., Benjamin Lebwohl, and Ruby Greywoode, 2015, "Celiac Disease," *The Journal of Al-*

lergy and Clinical Immunology, Vol. 135 No. 5, (May), pp. 1099–1106.

Grover, Steven A., Mohammed Kaouache, Philip Rempel, Lawrence Joseph, Martin Dawes, David C.W. Lau, and Ilka Lowensteyn, 2015, "Years of Life Lost and Healthy Life-Years Lost from Diabetes and Cardiovascular Disease in Overweight and Obese People: A Modelling Study," *The Lancet Diabetes & Endocrinology*, Vol. 3 No. 2, (February), pp. 114–122.

Guthrie, Katherine and Jan Sokolowsky, 2014, "Obesity and Household Financial Distress," *Critical Finance Review*, Forthcoming (October 14), 79 pp. Available at: http://ssrn.com/abstract=1786536.

Hall, Katherine S., Katherine D. Hoerster, and William S. Yancy, Jr., 2015, "Post-Traumatic Stress Disorder, Physical Activity, and Eating Behaviors," *Epidemiolic Reviews*, Vol. 37 No. 1, (January), pp. 103–115.

Helman, Ruth, Nevin Adams, Craig Copeland, and Jack VanDerhei, 2013, *The 2013 Retirement Confidence Survey: Perceived Savings Needs Outpace Reality for Many*, Employee Benefit Research Institute, Issue Brief No. 384, (March). Available at: http://www.ebri.org/pdf/surveys/rcs/2013/EBRI_IB _03-13.No384.RCS.pdf.

Helman, Ruth, Nevin Adams, Craig Copeland, and Jack VanDerhei, 2014, *The 2014 Retirement Confidence Survey: Confidence Rebounds—for Those With Retirement Plans*, Employee Benefit Research

Institute, Issue Brief No. 397, (March). Available at: http://www.ebri.org/pdf/surveys/rcs/2014/EBRI_IB _397_Mar14.RCS.pdf.

Helman, Ruth, Craig Copeland, and Jack Van-Derhei, 2015, *The 2015 Retirement Confidence Survey: Having a Retirement Savings Plan a Key Factor in Americans' Retirement Confidence*, Employee Benefit Research Institute, Issue Brief No. 413, (April). Available at: http://www.ebri.org/pdf/briefspdf/EBRI_IB_413_Apr 15_RCS-2015.pdf.

HHL, 2013, "Exercise is an all-natural treatment to fight depression," *Harvard Health Letter*, (August 1).

HMHL, 2010, "The Quirky Brain: Why Eating Slowly Helps Make People Feel Full," *Harvard Mental Health Letter*, Vol. 27 No. 4, (October), p. 7. Available at: http://www.health.harvard.edu/newsletters/Harvard_ Mental_Health_Letter/2010/October.

HSPH, 2012, "Food Pyramids and Plates: What Should You Really Eat?," Harvard School of Public Health, The Nutrition Source, Available at: http://www.hsph.harvard.edu/nutritionsource/pyram id-full-story/ (dated October 2012; downloaded July 2015).

HSPH, 2015, "Keep the Multi, Skip the Heavily Fortified Foods," Harvard School of Public Health, The Nutrition Source, Available at:

http://www.hsph.harvard.edu/nutritionsource/folic-acid/ (dated 2015; downloaded July 2015).

Jamrisko, Michelle, 2015, "Americans' Spending on Dining Out Just Overtook Grocery Sales for the First Time Ever," *Bloomberg News Online*, Available at: http://www.bloomberg.com/news/articles/2015-04-14/americans-spending-on-dining-out-just-overtook-grocery-sales-for-the-first-time-ever (dated April 15, 2015; downloaded July 2015).

Jordan, Lawrence A., 2002, *The Dirty Dozen: 12 Nasty Fighting Techniques for Any Self-Defense Situation*, Paladin Press: Boulder, CO, U.S.

Kell, John, 2015, "Diet Coke Sales Continue to Fizzle," *Fortune Magazine Online*, Available at: http://fortune.com/2015/04/22/diet-coke-sales-fizzle/ (dated April 22, 2015; downloaded July 2015).

Martínez, María Elena, Elizabeth T. Jacobs, John A. Baron, James R. Marshall, and Tim Byers, 2012, "Dietary Supplements and Cancer Prevention: Balancing Potential Benefits against Proven Harms," *Journal of the National Cancer Institute*, Vol. 104 No. 10, (May), pp. 732–739.

Neville, C.E., M.C. McKinley, V.A. Holmes, D. Spence, and J.V. Woodside, 2014, "The Relationship between Breastfeeding and Postpartum Weight Change: A Systematic Review and Critical Evaluation," *International Journal of Obesity*, Vol. 38 No. 4, (April), pp. 577–590.

NHS, 2011, Factsheet 4: Physical Activity Guidelines for Adults (19–64 Years). Available at: http://www.nhs.uk/Livewell/fitness/Documents/adults-19-64-years.pdf, 1 p.

Pagoto, Sherry L., Kristin L. Schneider, Jamie S. Bodenlos, Bradley M. Appelhans, Matthew C. Whited, Yunsheng Ma and Stephenie C. Lemon, 2012, "Association of Post-Traumatic Stress Disorder and Obesity in a Nationally Representative Sample," *Obesity*, Vol. 20 No. 1, (January), pp. 200–205.

Parkin, D.M., 2011, "Cancers Attributable to Reproductive Factors in the UK in 2010," *British Journal of Cancer*, Vol. 105 No. S2, (December), pp. S73-S76.

Parkin, D.M., and L. Boyd, 2011, "Cancers Attributable to Overweight and Obesity in the UK in 2010," *British Journal of Cancer*, Vol. 105 No. S2, (December), pp. S34-S37.

Parkin, D.M., L. Boyd, and L.C. Walker, 2011, "The Fraction of Cancer Attributable to Lifestyle and Environmental Factors in the UK in 2010," *British Journal of Cancer*, Vol. 105 No. S2, (December), pp. S77-S81.

Pereira, Greg F., Cynthia M. Bulik, Mark A. Weaver, Wesley C. Holland, and Timothy F. Platts-Mills, 2015, "Malnutrition among Cognitively Intact, Noncritically Ill Older Adults in the Emergency Department," *Annals of Emergency Medicine*, Vol. 65, No. 1, (January), pp. 85–91.

Pratt, Laura A., and Debra J. Brody, 2014, "Depression and Obesity in the U.S. Adult Household Population, 20052010," *NCHS Data Brief*, No. 167, (October), 8 pp.

Saslow, Debbie, 2013, "Can Breastfeeding Lower Breast Cancer Risk?," The American Cancer Society, Available at: http://www.cancer.org/cancer/news/expertvoices/post/2013/05/07/can-breastfeeding-lower-breast-cancer-risk.aspx, (dated May 7, 2013; downloaded July 2015).

SEC, 2012, "Investor Bulletin: Affinity Fraud," *Office of Investor Education and Advocacy: Investor Alert*, (September), 4 pp. Available at: http://www.sec.gov/investor/alerts/affinityfraud.pdf, (dated September 2012; downloaded August 2015).

Sharma, Andrea J., Deborah L. Dee, and Samantha M. Harden, 2014, "Adherence to Breastfeeding Guidelines and Maternal Weight 6 Years After Delivery," *Pediatrics*, Vol. 134 Supplement 1, (September 1), pp. S42–S49.

Su, Dada, Maria Pasalich, Andy H. Lee, and Colin W. Binns, 2013, "Ovarian Cancer Risk is Reduced by Prolonged Lactation: A Case-Control Study in Southern China," *American Journal of Clinical Nutrition*, Vol. 97 No. 2, (February), pp. 354–359.

Sugarman, Muriel, and Kathleen A. Kendall-Tackett, 1995, "Weaning Ages in a Sample of American Women

Who Practice Extended Breastfeeding," *Clinical Pediatrics*, Vol. 34 No. 12, (December), pp. 642–647.

U.S. Department of Health and Human Services, 1996, *Physical Activity and Health: A Report of the Surgeon General.* Atlanta, GA: U.S. Department of Health and Human Services, Centers for Disease Control and Prevention, National Center for Chronic Disease Prevention and Health Promotion.

Vanga, Rohini, and Daniel A. Leffler, 2013, "Gluten Sensitivity: Not Celiac and Not Certain," *Gastroenterology*, Vol. 145 No. 2, (August), pp. 276–279.

WCRF/AICR, 2007, "Food, Nutrition, Physical Activity, and the Prevention of Cancer: A Global Perspective," World Cancer Research Fund/American Institute for Cancer Research, Washington DC, 537 pp. Available at: http://www.dietandcancerreport.org/cancer_resource _center/downloads/Second_Expert_Report_full.pdf (dated November 2007; downloaded July 2015).

Index

www.ingramcontent.com/pod-product-compliance
Lightning Source LLC
Chambersburg PA
CBHW050129280326
41933CB00010B/1304